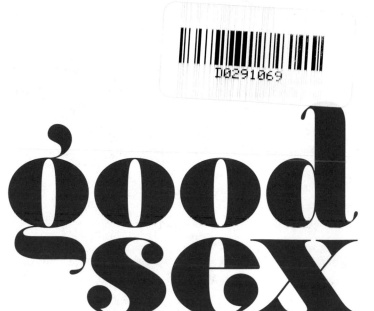

good sex

Getting Off without·Checking Out

JESSICA GRAHAM

North Atlantic Books
Berkeley, California

Published by
North Atlantic Books   Cover and book design by Debbie Berne
Berkeley, California   Printed in the United States of America

Good Sex: Getting Off without Checking Out is sponsored and published by the Society for the Study of Native Arts and Sciences (dba North Atlantic Books), an educational nonprofit based in Berkeley, California, that collaborates with partners to develop cross-cultural perspectives, nurture holistic views of art, science, the humanities, and healing, and seed personal and global transformation by publishing work on the relationship of body, spirit, and nature.

North Atlantic Books' publications are available through most bookstores. For further information, visit our website at www.northatlanticbooks.com or call 800-733-3000.

Library of Congress Cataloguing-in-Publication data is available from the publisher upon request.

ISBN: 9781623172343 (print) | ISBN: 9781623172350 (ebook)

1 2 3 4 5 6 7 8 9 United 22 21 20 19 18 17

Printed on recycled paper

praise for *good sex*

"Imagine the wisdom of meditation, the sexiness of truth, and the grace of vulnerability rolled into one joy-to-read book. This book is a treasure that will open your mind, awaken your heart, and ignite your body."

—Shauna L. Shapiro, PhD, author of *Mindful Discipline*

"An engaging, sincere, and insightful exploration that reveals how one can infuse sex with that magical 'something else' that we long for. Supported by numerous helpful exercises and practices to help you get there. Definitely a good read!"

—Diana Richardson, author of *The Heart of Tantric Sex; Tantric Orgasm for Women; Tantric Sex for Men*; and *Slow Sex*

"I can't imagine a person more qualified to write this book. Besides being a hardcore spiritual warrior, Jessica Graham has dedicated her life to exploring and understanding sexuality in all its forms."

—Michael Taft, author of *The Mindful Geek*

"A skilled mindfulness and meditation guide, Jessica Graham takes the deeply personal and spiritual art of mindfulness and shows us how it can be applied for massive change inside and out, and most importantly that sex should not be excluded but in fact is an integral part of that journey."

—Moushumi Ghose, MA, MFT, author of *Classic Sex Positions Reinvented*

"Mindfulness during sex means much more than banishing thoughts of the day or turning off your phone. Jessica Graham leads you through learning a meditative practice that enriches the connection with your partner and enhances your own sexual experience and the intensity of your orgasms. Even if you've never meditated before—or considered it! —Graham takes you step-by-step. Her candor about her own background makes this more than a self-help guide—it's a shared journey."

—Joan Price, author of *The Ultimate Guide to Sex after 50*

"Full of handy tips for exploring your sexuality and enhancing your pleasure."

—Lorin Roche, author of *The Radiance Sutras*

"In a world that shows us distorted views of sex and distracts from inner inquiry in general, Jessica's work clearly illustrates sex is truly a mindfulness practice.... [Her] willingness to be vulnerable makes *Good Sex* accessible and useful."

—Nicole Daedone, author of *Slow Sex*

"Hidden within the colorful, fragrant, silky petals of physical love, lies a subtle treasure that transcends sensuality ... Jessica is eminently qualified to point people to this jewel in the lotus, and *Good Sex* connects the dots."

—Shinzen Young, author of *The Science of Enlightenment*

"In *Good Sex*, Jessica Graham offers clear, compassionate, and provocative instruction for integrating mindfulness and sexuality. *Good Sex* offers insight on how to use the dynamic realm of sexuality as a laboratory for mindfulness. This book is deep, accessible, kind, clear, edgy, and experiential. It is meant to inspire and ignite possibility in a world that still holds the illusion of a sex-spirit divide."

—Deborah Eden Tull, Zen teacher, founder of Mindful Living Revolution, and author of *Relational Mindfulness: Reclaiming Our Shared Power in an Age of Disconnect*

To the DJ of Life.

You are a goddamn warrior.

I love you.

You must love in such a way that the person
you love feels free.

—Thich Nhat Hanh

Sex is always about emotions. Good sex is about
free emotions; bad sex is about blocked emotions.

—Deepak Chopra

A lot of people are afraid to say what they want.
That's why they don't get what they want.

—Madonna

contents

acknowledgments

Tim McKee, Alison Knowles, Bevin Donahue and the entire NAB Team—thank you for giving my book such a great home.

Maggie Marr

Debbie Berne

Christine Rose Elle

Jennifer Kamenetz

Rachel Neumann

Jacob Surpin

Lorraine Clark

Terri Saul

Shauna Shapiro

Hisae Matsuda

Shayan Asgharnia

Miranda July

Sarah Drescher

Louis C. Oberlander

Johnny Camacho

Margie Woods

Leslie Herrick

Gia Esquivel

Andreas Panosyan

Jennifer Howd

The Eastside Mindfulness Collective

Tristan Taormino

Ada Douglass

The Kirk-Dacker Family

Clark D. Schaefer

Richard Grossinger

Casey Marie Fischer and all the brave, beautiful, and sexy ladies of In Bed In LA.

David Schnarch, Ph.D. for writing *Passionate Marriage*.

My teachers, healers, and guides: Ellen Murphy, Susan Coates, Arnold McMahon, Kimberly Ann Johnson, Joshua Bitton, Jenoa Harlow, Dafna Laurie, Elizabeth Bast, Lindsay Frame, Shinzen Young, Saul Kotzubei, Adyashanti, Mukti, Greg Beckett, Lee Ann Teaney, Erin Smith, Alan Padula, Moushumi Ghose, and all the rest.

All my students and clients for inspiring me to keep growing no matter what.

My mom, Linda Clark, for reading to me, putting creativity first, and raising me to know that I could have spots *and* stripes.

My sisters Dian and Melanie, and my brother Sam. The thought of you guys chases any loneliness away.

All my lovers, past, present, and future.

Stella De Mont for being the best Best Friend ever. My Little One loves your Little One.

Tracy McMillan, for being your amazing and inspiring self and helping me to be mine. Thank you for ALL you do. You are instrumental in my evolution.

acknowledgments

Michael Taft for introducing me to the writer inside of me, believing in me every step of the way, and of course, for destroying my life. This book would not exist without you.

Christopher Kelly, for loving me with such bravery and kindness. Thank you for inspiring me to always aim just slightly past my edge. Thank you for being the catalyst that launched me into the woman who could write this book. Thank you for being my man. I love you.

This book is for you.

It's for you in whatever kind of body you live in.
It's for you in whatever way you express your sexuality.
It's for you in whatever gender you identify with—
and it's for you if you don't identify with any gender at all.
It's for you in whatever way you choose to be in
romantic relationships.

This book is for you.

one

the adventure begins

I have been in the trenches. I know what it is like to squeeze my eyes shut during sex and hope that my partner is doing the same, terrified of seeing or being seen. I know what it is like to be able to "relax" and ask for what I really want only when I'm drunk. I know what it's like to only be attracted to people who don't treat me all that well. To feel more alone during sex. To have sex with someone I don't even like. To wonder if my spiritual life will ever spill over into my sex life. I know how it feels to be told that my sexuality is wrong. I know the sound of me faking an orgasm. I know the feeling that there must be something more.

I have been there.

Somewhere along the way, I decided to make a change in my life. Now I know what it is to turn on the lights and look directly into my partner's eyes as I come. I no longer need alcohol to help me relax or communicate. I have tools for working through periods of low sex drive. I can allow myself to be loved, respected, and treated with loving kindness. I know how to fully embody my pleasure, free from thoughts and anxiety. I now have a relationship that engages my sexual expression and is based on honesty and love. My

1

spiritual life and sex life are interconnected. I don't allow the fears or judgments of others to dictate my sexual expression. I never, ever fake it. I have found that sexual discovery is endless.

Of course, I haven't been *exactly* where you've been. We all have our own unique experiences in life and with sex. Sexuality is different for everyone, and the tools in this book are meant to be flexible, to suit different people. I will share my story with you and what I have learned, with the knowledge that life is a constant process of learning and evolving. Not everything in this book will resonate with everyone. I do invite you to open your mind to what lies beyond your current comfort zone and adopt a stance of openness on this journey.

Sitting down and practicing meditation every day reengineered my whole life, including my sex life. It wasn't only meditation, of course: I also incorporated therapy, recovery groups, bodywork, writing, and reading into my practice. But meditation has been the bedrock from which my sexual awakening has sprung.

This book will give you the tools to start a meditation practice, if you would like one, or deepen your practice if you already have one. After that, the next step is to bring mindfulness into your sex life. Sexual awakening isn't a spectator sport; it requires some work, and this book will guide you through the process. There will be plenty of fun along the way, though. Waking up can be an amazing adventure.

Bringing mindfulness into sex invites you to open yourself to a bigger, richer, and more present life. If we put our sexuality in a shoebox under the bed, we are putting a part of ourselves in there too. Every present moment, if we bring our full attention to it, is a chance to wake up. Awakening can happen while you load the dishwasher or while you press your lover's body against a wall and make her scream with pleasure. As you bring more mindfulness to your lovemaking, you can get a glimpse of your own brand of enlightenment. These moments of awakening that come from deeply experiencing sex add up. You may find that the intense connection you feel with your partner during sex extends to include the whole world.

I have an old friend with whom I reconnected several years ago. The first few times we hung out she spent a good deal of time sharing with me how much I had changed since we had been teenagers. Of course, most people do change during the years between sixteen and thirty-something. She reminded me how wild and reckless I had been. She told me of all the escapades I had led: adventurous tales of skinny-dipping in stranger's pools and streaking in suburban neighborhoods. There were also darker tales of close calls with drunk driving and mornings of regret from the night before.

It was a huge surprise to my friend that I was teaching people how to bring spirituality into their sex lives. "You told me you were totally over sex when you were fifteen!" she said. I had only a vague memory of saying something like that, but she was sure of it. She recounted my tight jaw and stony words like it was yesterday. She told me that she had felt sad for me, being so jaded at such a young age. While I love who I am today, and all those experiences led me to this point, I felt a little grief hearing about that teenage version of me.

The Long and Winding Road to Good Sex

It started in the back seat of a green Chevrolet Chevelle, with an eighteen-year-old with tattoos and a ponytail. It was a chilly night in May, at a graduation party out in the woods of Eastern Pennsylvania. I was just fourteen, wearing my favorite flannel shirt and cutoffs. I had made a promise to my mom that I wouldn't drink that night, but not that I wouldn't get high. I smoked a joint and I set out on a mission. Tonight was the night. I would lose my virginity, come hell or high water.

The guy with the ponytail had been my crush all year and seemed like a good candidate. I noticed that he had his eye on another girl that night. I was relieved when she left early and he turned his gaze to me. He asked me to take a walk with him, and that walk ended in the back seat of his car. Right before he reached up to the glove box to get a condom he asked, "You wanna do this?" Afterward, when retelling the story to my friends, I changed this to, "Are you sure you want to do this? We don't have to if you aren't ready." I wanted him to seem more considerate. Looking back, I do appreciate that he asked for consent. That's more than I can say for a few other men I've been with.

I kept my turquoise All-Star high tops on the whole time. It hurt a lot but didn't go on for long. Afterward I told him that I'd remember that night for a long time. He lit a cigarette and said that we should head back to the party. I had never even made out with anyone before. I was high and remember that night as if I was far away. I just did it because I thought it had to be done; it didn't really matter if I was actually present for it. Later that year, I had sex again: this time in a field with a twenty-year-old, also with a ponytail. I was intoxicated again.

This pattern went on for many years, sex without presence or intimacy, though not always with older men with ponytails. Not always with men. What remained the same was my inability to really be conscious for sexual experiences. Even if I wasn't drunk or high, I was checked out in some way. I didn't look into my lover's eyes. I was lost in my own mind, needing a fantasy to climax. I didn't feel a sense of merging or the sacred. Sex was all about checking out and getting off.

By my late twenties, these patterns had driven me to an all-time low. I had been drinking since I was twelve and still depended on drugs and alcohol to get me through tough times. My patterns in relationships had led me to a partner who was verbally and emotionally abusive, but I was unable to leave. I started thinking about ending my life. I spent a whole day wandering around Hollywood trying to find a crisis center that would take me. That day was a wake-up call. It was time to make a change.

I began by getting sober and committed to a year of celibacy and being relationship-free. I wanted to break the old patterns and create new ones. When you clear out old patterns, you create space for new ways of living. The new pattern that changed my life more than any other was my daily meditation practice.

Waking Up

After I had been sober a little over a year, I started dating a kind and loving man. It was the first truly healthy relationship I had ever been in and it primed me to have a whole new kind of romantic partnership. While I was still shut down sexually in some ways, the sex we had was the most conscious and mindful I had had up to that point. That relationship didn't work out long-term, but it was an important one for me, and I credit him with inspiring me to get serious about meditation.

Early in our relationship, my new boyfriend started hosting a meditation group at his house. It wasn't until the teacher, Michael W. Taft, accused me of being "chicken," that I actually tried it out. At my very first meditation session I saw that I could maintain separation from my thoughts, even when my thoughts were going crazy. I was full of anxiety that day about a job I was hoping to get. During the meditation, I watched those anxious thoughts come and go. I was a witness to them, rather than being stuck inside of my monkey mind. This was a revelation for me.

I dove into my meditation practice, and so began a series of awakenings that rocked my world. My practice showed me that I was not my thoughts or emotions. I'd heard spiritual teachers say "You are not your mind," and now I knew it to be true. With this insight, I was able to explore the wild mystery of what I really am. I started to realize how interconnected everything is: There was no illusion of separation anymore. It became hard to think of myself as a solid and fixed thing, as I had done before. There was no one me, but instead a constant flow of experience that made up infinite selves. I fell in love with life, each tiny seemingly mundane thing. I laugh now when I tell people how I cradled my water bottle with total love and adoration after a particularly intense experience of absolute love in a meditation.

In my early practice I had many of these "peak experiences." Some of them were deep states of blissful concentration, and some were full on sixties-style acid trips. While some of these peak states were coupled with deep insights, others were due more to the intensity of my practice and my personal history (and are in no way necessary for everyone). Some of these states were exhilarating, and some were terrifying. As I began to process years of pent up emotion, my subconscious had some frightening displays for me. But I got the good stuff too. The flashy experiences helped motivate me to keep meditating, but eventually they slowed down. As my practice took on a calmer and more grounded tone, I began to see the results of my hard work. My relationships began to change with my family, my friends, and my partner. Most importantly, I started to see a clear choice in front of me: Did I want to suffer, or take another path?

About a year into my meditation practice, my father became very ill. He was an alcoholic, and when he got hit with cancer he couldn't stop drinking or smoking. He wasted away. He and I had a profoundly deep but also complex and challenging relationship. We were often called "Twin Flames" because we looked and acted so much alike. He was one of my very best friends, which was wonderful, but also meant that he became my drinking buddy when I was only fourteen. We took trips together, stared up at the night sky together, got drunk together, and sat in the car listening to The Rolling Stones, The Eagles, and Led Zeppelin together.

As I got older, I tried to become more responsible: I tried to drink less and spend more time working and less time playing. This caused me to grow apart from my dad. I no longer wanted to be around him when he was drunk. I found his alcoholism embarrassing and depressing. But our special connection never faded. I remember one night after I had been living in Los Angeles for a number of years, I was watching some obscure film that I had rented. Just as the credits started to roll, my dad called me from Philadelphia to tell me about this film he thought I should see. It was the same one I had just finished. That kind of synchronicity was commonplace for us.

At a certain point in his illness, it became clear that he wasn't going to get better. At first, I was scared to buy a one-way ticket and be with him until he died. But eventually I knew I had to go. Armed with my practice, I sat by his side for the last month of his life with love, compassion, and acceptance for him and for myself. I administered his medications, and at the end, I even changed his diapers. I didn't judge him for his alcoholism anymore. Hell, I put beer in his feeding tube when he asked me to. The day before he died, he was so underweight that I could pick him up in my arms like a baby. That last day and evening I washed his body, whispered to him everything I hadn't yet said, meditated on his face, and listened to his heartbeat until it became faint. Along with my mom, my sisters, a cat, and dog, I stood beside his bed as he took his last breath. I held his socked feet as his frail and broken body finally let go.

Without my meditation practice, that experience would have been much different. I would have been so full of anger, resentment, and grief that I wouldn't have been able to offer the care that I did. That one year of meditation healed and prepared me for my father's death in a way that nothing else could have.

Not long after my dad died, one of my meditation teachers suggested that I start teaching meditation. Soon I was sharing my experience with groups and individuals. In the beginning I primarily taught mindfulness, focusing on learning to witness thoughts and emotions. That type of technique had changed my life and I wanted to spread the good word. I had found a new calling, but I still had a lot to learn when it came to integrating my spiritual life with my sex life.

Although my spiritual growth had taken off, I had yet to take a hard look at my sex life. I was still cut off from my body during sex. I still failed to fully connect with my partners. I did enjoy sex, but I was only scraping the surface. I had no idea what good sex was. Good sex invites you to be fully present for every single sweet drop of pleasure.

I was only partially present for my partners because I was only partially present for myself. I tended to attract people who matched my own emotional and spiritual evolution. Very few of my partners ever called me out on disappearing during sex, because they did as well. My meditation practice, however, alerted me to my disappearance. Observing my thoughts and emotions every day in formal meditation was revealing the parts of me that were hidden away.

There was a woman inside of me waking up. She wanted a new kind of sex, passion, and pleasure. She wanted to explore the far reaches of her sexuality and beyond. She wanted to feel a lover truly become one with her. The awakening I was having in other areas couldn't help but spill over into my sex life. I wanted more. My authentic sexuality was bursting forth.

Around this time, I read *Passionate Marriage*, by David Schnarch, PhD. I was struck by his writing about looking into your partner's eyes while you climax.[1] At first I thought, *No way. Never going to happen.* The idea of seeing and being seen at that vulnerable moment made my skin crawl. But I was committed to allowing my sexuality to shine and slowly began to take a peek at my partners during sex. There wasn't any eye contact yet, but it was progress for me.

It took time to go from the desire for good sex to actually having good sex. I had to work through years of old habits. And there was another hold up: I didn't have partners who wanted to practice mindful sex. Why would I? Up until then, the idea of mindful sex frightened me. So I had to be patient. It was frustrating to be ready for a new kind of sex but not have the tools or the willing partner with whom to take the next step. Luckily, my meditation practice helped me hang out in the gray area without suffering too much.

I began seeing a sex therapist, and he invited me to find ways to sexually heal and blossom without a partner. This was such a valuable piece of advice for me. I could start practicing mindful sex on my own. I began to read more about sex: instructional manuals, erotic fiction, and personal essays. I meditated on the feelings of rejection and disappointment I felt when partners didn't want to try a new way of lovemaking. I bought sexy underwear and red lipstick and spent time seducing myself. I brought mindfulness into masturbation, exploring and finding new kinds of pleasure.

I worked a lot on sexual trauma and negative sexual beliefs. I also dove into my creative life: writing, drawing, dancing, and acting. I found that sexual energy and creative energy were the same thing and could enhance and inspire the other. In short, I made my sexual awakening a priority.

I've come to learn, based on my own experience and that of my friends and students, that when you focus your attention on an area of your life, it will change. My sexuality was no exception. It sounds cliché, but during the first wave of my own sexual revolution, I took on a glow. My friends asked what was going on, my classes grew, and I became more playful and light. I had access to more energy than ever before.

The first time I looked into a lover's eyes while we made love was frightening, exhilarating. It was, in essence, a new first time. Madonna's "Like a Virgin" comes to mind when I remember it. There was a sincerity and openness that I had never felt. It was also obvious that, of course, this is the way it should be. I began to have profound spiritual experiences during sex. I was actually "becoming one" with my partner. We were connected in a way that I had never been with anyone before. And it was fun! Sex became both spiritual and an adult playground. I started to have more flexibility in what aroused me. I discovered new pleasures and fantasies. It was a meditation in action that I had never known. As a result, my creative life began to expand too. I found that I had more energy to write, act, draw, and play.

My relationships benefitted as well. I was no longer hiding from my partners. I was present, vulnerable, and open. My body became incredibly sensitive. I could feel things that I hadn't even known existed. With this greater connection to my own body, I connected with my partners on a much deeper level.

What is possible to share with another person continues to shock and delight me. Now that I'm not cut off from such an important aspect of myself, I have so much more to offer my partner. I also have more to offer as a teacher. Being a teacher means modeling the willingness to keep growing. If I left my sexuality unexplored and stayed checked out, I'd be limiting my ability to be of service as a teacher.

I've been teaching since 2009. I started by facilitating a small group in Los Angeles once a week that has since grown into a flourishing community called The Eastside Mindfulness Collective. Several teachers lead weekly classes, both online and in person, as well as hold workshops and events. I teach everyday awakening through mindfulness and inquiry techniques. I give raw, down-to-earth talks on being human. In addition to my classes and workshops, I offer private sessions to individuals, couples, and families. I also teach for other organizations and special events in the Los Angeles area and beyond. In recent years, I have expanded my teaching to include my work with mindful sex. I'm deeply in love with this area of my work. It's such a joyful experience to see someone awaken sexually.

Sex is such a big part of being human, yet it is often ignored in discussions of spiritual practice and awakening. This is why I have focused my efforts on using my experience to help others. To wake up fully, we need to invite awakening into all parts of our lives—including our sex lives.

I had another therapist who said: "As you get older, sex gets weird." He was a longtime meditation practitioner and a very awake person. I took what he said to mean that when you continue to bring mindfulness to sex, you access deeper and deeper mysterious layers. Over the years, my sexuality has changed and changed and changed again. Sometimes it *does* get weird, in a delightful way. When I greet sex with openness and acceptance, the possibilities are endless.

A couple of weeks back my partner and I had a few hours free, and decided to use the time for a sexual adventure. We spoke openly and with joyful laughter about what we might explore. There was a sense of fun, excitement, and total trust as we stopped talking and started undressing each other. Before long I was all tied up and not going anywhere.

I won't get into the rest of the intimate details, but I will share the most important detail: I was present for every moment of our sexcapade. I felt it all, and so did my partner.

Mindful Sex

Having mindful sex doesn't mean always making love while staring into your partner's eyes, and whispering sweet nothings. "Mindful" doesn't mean mushy or boring. In my experience, mindful sex can be dirty, fun, exciting, and even rough (mindful sex can absolutely involve handcuffs). It is based on who you are in that moment.

Mindful sex is not perfect sex. If you are stuck in an ideal, you miss out on what is happening in the moment. So many deny themselves spectacular sex because they are caught up in how they think it should be. Your sexuality is a gift that you get to unwrap again and again throughout your life. It changes and evolves just like your body does, just like nature does, just like everything does. This book isn't meant to give you a cookie-cutter sex life. Instead, it's an invitation to venture into the mystery and beauty of your authentic sexuality. By simply being present with yourself and your partner while you are having sex, you can connect in ways that seem magical. It's not actually magic: It's how life is when you show up for it.

As you begin this adventure, remember that ultimately you are your own best teacher. My experience and suggestions are just a jumping off point. As you get to know your body and begin to gain some perspective on the stories in your mind, a new kind of wisdom will emerge. A wisdom that you can trust to lead you skill-fully through your sex life and beyond. No one can give you this wisdom; you must find it for yourself. So take what you like from this book and leave the rest. One size does not fit all.

I don't believe in one true answer for sex issues, but I do know that adding mindfulness to sex yields results. I hope to empower you to find your own path to mindful sex. We are going to explore everything from those dreaded open-eyed orgasms, to non-monogamy, to trauma. I will continue to share details of my story with you, uncensored. What better way to make use of all my trials and errors than to share them to help you?

It's incredibly important to let go of getting this right. There is no right way. If you have a firm idea of how your sex *should* be, it's time to let go of that. This is an adventure and an exploration, not a contest. Cast out the desire to be the best at mindful sex or the best at meditation, and just be here now. As you let go of your expec-tations and ego-laced goals, you will wake up to reality. When you truly reside in reality, your experience will blow any fantasy out of the water. You'll begin to see how limitless life actually is.

A note for my trans, gender-fluid, and gender-nonconforming readers. I am a cisgender female and most of my sexual experiences are with cisgender men and women. At this point I also have very few experiences sharing my mindful sex work with members of the trans or gender-nonconforming community. While that is the knowledge base I am coming from, I do my best in this book to make the writing accessible to everyone. There may be times when you have to trans-late the material a bit, but know that this book is for you too.

I use the words "penis" and "vagina" in this book. Feel free to cross out those words and add pussy, cock, vajaja, wiener, cunt, dick, honeypot, joystick, or whatever tickles your fancy. I know some of the words I just listed can be offensive to some, whereas for others penis and vagina can seem awkward or too formal. Call your genitalia by any name you like.

Another word I use in this book is "fucking." Dr. Schnarch uses this word in *Passionate Marriage*,[2] and I'm doing the same. I've come to know fucking as a very different thing than "making love." They both have their place in good sex and have different intellectual and behavioral meanings depending on who you are. If the word fucking freaks you out, feel free to replace it as you wish. I do recommend that you explore what fucking versus making love means to you. Is it possible that you have never experienced what fucking at its best can be? This is worth a little mindful investigation.

You will see me mention trauma many times throughout this book. I am incredibly passionate about healing my own trauma and helping others heal theirs. Trauma recovery has been a huge part of my spiritual path and my personal healing. Toward the end of the book, I'll be delving much deeper into the subject of trauma with both my personal experiences and what I've seen as a teacher. I offer a little warning at the beginning of chapters that may be triggering for some.

Without a dedicated meditation practice, I would most likely still be sexually checked out. Just reading this book will not magically transform your sex life—you will need to put the practice of mindfulness into action. The next two chapters of this book are a mini-manual for mindfulness meditation. These are techniques that I teach in my classes, many inspired by Shinzen Young's mindfulness teachings.[3] Don't feel you need to retain all the information on the first read. Think of this as a reference that you can flip to at any time. I will refer to these techniques throughout the book.

Learning to have more mindful sex can bring up a lot of emotions. This is especially true for anyone who is working through sexual trauma. It is important that you get a lot of support along the way, and just meditating may not cut it. A good therapist, recovery groups, and a spiritual or meditation coach can be a huge help when delving into mindful sex. Take care of yourself and be patient and loving with whatever comes up. In this book we will explore ways to use meditation and mindfulness to address trauma and the shame that often accompanies it. That has been a big part of my story, and I'm honored to share what I have learned with you. I consider myself a spiritual person and this book has a spiritual tone. If even the word spiritual rubs you the wrong way, fear not. You can ignore that aspect of the book. Mindful sex does not have to fall into the spiritual category if that doesn't work for you. But don't throw the baby out with the bathwater. Try the practices for yourself and then decide if mindful sex is for you. Even if you do consider yourself to be spiritual, don't just take my word for it. This is your adventure. See for yourself what mindful sex can do for you. This path is uncharted. It's made of your experience, unfolding moment by moment, breath by breath, touch by touch. A willingness to dive into the present is all you need to begin your journey.

two

mindfulness manual: obstacles, faqs, and tips

Mindfulness meditation has been practiced for thousands of years. The Buddha taught his followers how to meditate on the breath, physical sensations, emotions, and thoughts way before mindfulness became the wildly popular word it is today. It's a tried and true practice that has stood the test of time.

Mindfulness is the practice of greeting all experiences with acceptance and curiosity. It allows you to know what you are feeling when you are feeling it and what you are thinking when you are thinking it. Mindfulness opens up a small space before acting on a thought. It's a path that allows you to stop resisting what is and embrace the present moment. Being mindful helps you to create a new relationship with your emotions, mind, and the world at large. Meditation is a formal practice that you carve out time for each day. There are many different types of meditation from many different traditions. In this book we will be primarily focusing on mindfulness meditation, traditionally called *vipassana*, which means to see things as they really are. We will also explore loving kindness or Mettā practice, as well as many special exercises aimed at bringing more mindfulness into your sex life.

I've put together a collection of some of my favorite techniques to get you started. Most of these techniques are based on or inspired by Shinzen Young's mindfulness teachings.[1] Throughout the book, I'll refer to these techniques and offer ways to use them in your sex life. Don't feel that you have to master all of these techniques. Choose the ones that seem most interesting and apply them to what you are addressing in your life.

Frequent Obstacles to Starting a Meditation Practice

Many people have heard about meditation before, and might even believe in the benefits of a regular meditation practice, but have found reasons to stop themselves from incorporating meditation into their daily lives. I understand that struggle: Meditation can seem like a big and frightening commitment. Before we go into specific meditation practices and techniques, let's address a few reasons for not meditating that you may be holding on to.

I can't meditate because my mind is too noisy.

You do not have to have a quiet mind to meditate. I always tell new students that meditation isn't about getting rid of our thoughts, it's about creating a new relationship with them.

Let me share this story with you. A group of monks from the Forest Thai tradition were sitting around, asking their teacher, Ajahn Chah, some questions. One asked, "What kind of person has no thoughts?" They threw around some guesses: an enlightened being? A Buddha? Ajahn Chah looked at them and simply said, "A dead person."

We are living humans! We have living brains that think thoughts. If you don't understand that basic condition, you are in for a very frustrating meditation experience. There are times when our minds quiet down—usually when we are deeply immersed in something (perhaps when working an art project, playing a sport, or having sex). Meditation, of course, can help with reaching these more "quiet" states. As you start to practice, you'll find that the mind settles over time, especially during longer sits or on meditation retreats. It's a wonderful feeling to be free from thought, but thought will always return. That's because you're alive. Freedom from thought comes not in the absence of thought, but in cultivating a new relationship to your thoughts and feelings. That's what meditation is about.

I don't have time to meditate.

Yes, you do. Unless you never watch Netflix; do any nonwork-related social networking, obsessively empty your inbox to get to zero new messages; or read, watch, or listen to news of any kind, you have time. You have a lot more time than you think you do. You have ten minutes a day for your meditation practice. You'll just need to start the new habit, and maybe let go of some old ones.

There are also lots of ways to bring your meditation practice into your life off the cushion. We will explore some ways to do that in this chapter.

I live in the city, and the street sounds are too loud for me to be able to meditate.

Who said you needed a noiseless environment to meditate? If it's noisy, that's just something to accept. Keep returning to your meditation and notice how your thoughts or sensations are affected by the sounds.

Sound is actually a wonderful thing to meditate on. I'm not including this technique in the manual, but it's very simple. Just listen to the sound. If you are pulled into thoughts about sounds, bring your attention back to the pure sound.

I can't meditate because I'm not religious, or even spiritual.

Meditation does not have to be religious or spiritual. Let go of that excuse. I am not religious, and I'm a meditation teacher! I do tend to talk in spiritual terms, but I don't subscribe to any particular spiritual philosophy or doctrine, and I won't ask you to either. If the more spiritual parts of this book or mentions of religion bother you, just skip those sections or read them with a snarky smirk. You can think of these practices as exercises for your mind. These practices will sharpen your concentration skills, give you more emotional flexibility, help you to understand other people better, and improve your sex life.

If you do follow a certain religion, that is also not a problem. Most religions have some form of contemplation already worked in. What you learn in this book can be a complement to the practices your religion already offers.

Meditation FAQs

If you are new to meditation, you probably have some questions. These are the most frequent ones that I've heard.

How often should I meditate?

Every day. This is pretty much a nonnegotiable. You will only receive the benefits of a meditation practice if you actually practice.

I've had private students who only want to practice when I'm there guiding them. They may gain some insight or experience some relaxation during our sessions, but they aren't able to carry those insights into their daily lives. In those situations, I'm really just a Band-Aid. For some people, reading spiritual self-help books like this one can work the same way. It would be like having a box full of books about learning French, but never trying to speak a word. So please practice, because the real healing and growth comes when you begin to make meditation a daily habit. Of course you'll miss a day here and there. I do too! The trick is to get back on track the next day, without making a big deal of the missed day or judging yourself.

How long should I meditate?

Ideally, thirty to sixty minutes a day, but I know this is not feasible for a lot of people. Ten minutes a day is a great start. Over time you'll be able to build it up. And remember that you probably have more time than you think you do.

Where and when should I meditate?

Wherever and whenever! For some people it can be helpful to choose a time of day (a lot of my students like to meditate in the morning) and a specific spot to meditate consistently. The routine can be helpful, especially in the beginning, in remembering to meditate every day.

It's nice to create a little area in your home that's just for meditation. You can keep your meditation chair or cushion there, along with anything that inspires you to practice. But having a specific place where you meditate isn't a requirement.

Do I need to face a certain direction,
light candles and incense, or say a special prayer?

Nope. All that's required is some uninterrupted time and you. Of course if a candle or a prayer is going to facilitate your practice, then go for it. This is your practice, your adventure. Make it work for you.

How do I prepare to meditate?

Let whoever you live with know that you are going to meditate (this translates to, "Don't bug me for the next fifteen minutes"). Put your phone on silent, and make sure your computer won't be tweeting at you either. Set a timer. I use the timer on my phone, but if you'd rather keep your phone out of the mix, get yourself a cheap digital kitchen timer. If you have a bad "phone checking" habit, the urge to sneak a peek might be too strong if it's nearby. Once your timer is set, settle into your posture and begin.

Posture

Your meditation posture is a personal thing, and you get to do what is best for your body. It's not necessary to sit in a full lotus position to meditate—in fact, you can meditate lying down! My style of sitting is usually half lotus, but that can change depending on how my body feels. Here are a few options for posture.

Sitting on the Floor

Sit cross-legged, in half lotus, or in full lotus (only if this is something you can do without excessive pain) on a cushion. Zafus are a special type of cushion made for meditation. You can find them in many online stores. Make sure that your butt is lifted up a bit on the cushion and that your pelvis is pointing down. This will help take some pressure off of your back. Either way, you may also want a blanket or cushioned mat (*zabuton*) under you as well. You don't need these special meditation props to meditate, but they can make the experience more comfortable.

Kneeling on a Bench

For some people using a meditation bench is a better option. These can also easily be purchased online. You sit on the bench with your legs folded under, kneeling on the floor. You will want a small cushion on the bench and some padding, like a blanket, under your knees.

Sitting in a Chair

Sitting in a chair is a great option if the floor doesn't work for you. There is absolutely no shame in using a chair. I have a friend who has had serious ongoing back issues. At her first meditation retreat she tried her best to sit on the floor, but the pain got worse and worse. She decided that she just wasn't going to be able to stick it out with this whole "meditate for ten days" thing. Finally, she told a teacher what was going on and the teacher laughed, saying, "Just sit on a chair, silly!" She now goes to meditation retreats regularly and happily meditates in a chair.

For this posture you'll want both feet on the ground. Don't cross your legs. Sit a bit away from the back of the chair or put cushions behind you, so that you don't slouch.

Whichever sitting version you use, imagine there is a balloon attached to a cord that starts at the base of your spine and runs all the way up and out of the top of your head. As your spine straightens, allow your body to relax. This is a gentle stacking of the spine; it shouldn't be rigid or tight. Allow your shoulders to drop down and back, and let go of any intentional tension in your body. Just use the muscles you need for sitting up. Allow everything else to relax as much as possible.

Lying Down

If sitting for an extended time is not possible for you due to an injury or chronic issue, you can always practice meditation lying down. The only problem with this posture is that it's very easy to fall asleep. So that is something you'll need to be aware of, because sleeping is not the same as meditating.

For the lying down posture, simply lie flat on the floor. This is just like *savasana* (corpse pose) at the end of a yoga class. Turn your palms up and allow your legs and feet to splay out. If you have lower back issues, try putting a pillow or rolled up blanket under your knees. Allow your whole body to melt into the ground. And stay awake.

Stillness

Once you are settled in, aim to sit still for your entire meditation. At first that can seem impossible, but as you practice it becomes easier. Moving around a bunch doesn't really help anyway. It's like Whack a Mole. You'll find that once you shift your posture because of an ache in your leg, you notice another ache somewhere else.

Your feet and legs may fall asleep—that's something you get used to. It's going to happen from time to time if you sit on the floor. After years of meditating, it generally doesn't bother me when my legs fall asleep. Sometimes I won't even realize until I try to stand up and I can't! I can also report that I've had no bodily damage due to sitting with some pins and needles.

This doesn't mean you are condemned to total motionlessness. You are *aiming* for stillness. When you become aware of the desire to move, pause. Take a moment to feel the discomfort and notice how emotions and thoughts arise in reaction to it. Being comfortable with discomfort can be incredibly helpful in life. If you still feel that you must move, then go ahead and move. Do your best to make the adjustment with as much mindfulness as you can. Move with intention, rather than compulsively. Pay attention to how it feels to move and how you feel after moving.

Often, a lot of the pain beginning meditators feel is a kind of emotional pain and resistance. It can be scary to sit with yourself—who knows what will come up? This type of pain is tricky and you'll have to explore to find out if that's what is going on for you. You might be sitting there with loads of pain, and then as soon as the timer goes off, the pain vanishes. As your body learns that it's safe to be still, this type of pain will subside.

There most likely will be some aches, pains, and pins and needles no matter how you sit. Even lying still can be uncomfortable at times. Noticing how uncomfortable it is to be still is often one of the first insights people have. Over time you will get accustomed to stillness and the pain will subside, and when it does arise it won't bother you as much. But please always listen to your own body and never push yourself to hold a posture that is causing extreme discomfort.

Relaxing from Your Head to Your Feet

After you have settled into your chosen posture, take a few minutes to relax. This period of relaxation is part of your meditation, and is included in the amount of time you've decided to practice. Don't worry if you can't relax completely. Just relax wherever you can. If there is tension that just doesn't want to loosen up, relax all around the tension, offering it acceptance. You may be amazed or overwhelmed by how much tension you discover. Do your best to keep inviting relaxation and focus on what is relaxed.

I always say that relaxing is a brave thing to do. We have tension in our bodies for all kinds of reasons. Some of us have been tense for a long time. A car accident or an emotional or physical trauma can create tension in the body. As we learn to relax we may come in contact with a lot of resistance and some challenging emotions. Over time your body will learn that it's okay to relax, and the years of trapped tension will begin to unwind.

I also recommend that you finish each session with a period of relaxation. You can include this in the timed session or just take thirty seconds to a minute after the timer goes off to relax your body.

Give it a try now. The instructions below can guide you through a relaxation exercise.

- Start at your forehead. Invite your forehead to soften and smooth out. Relax your eyebrows and the space between your eyebrows. Allow any expression to melt away.

- Relax your eyes and all the little muscles around your eyes. We tend to hold a lot of tension in the eyes, so take your time to allow them to relax.

- Relax down your cheeks and into your jaw. Invite the jaw to relax completely. Let the mouth drop open a little. If it feels good, very gently press your tongue into the roof of your mouth.

- Relax your neck and down into your shoulders. Let your shoulders drop down and back, allowing your chest to open slightly. Feel that relaxation move down your arms to your hands.

- Relax your chest and into your stomach. Invite the sides of your torso to relax.

- Relax your back, from the upper back all the way down to the lower back. Just use the muscles you need for sitting up and allow everything else to relax.

- Now invite your butt, hips, and pelvic area to relax. Soften the perineum. That is the space between your genitals and your anus.

- Relax down both of your legs. Relax your feet.

That's it. For some people, using visualization helps. You can imagine each muscle relaxing. Or you can visualize a warm golden liquid spreading through your body as you relax more and more.

It can also be helpful to start with a few deep breaths, sighing out loud on the exhale. If you are feeling particularly tense, you might want to try intentionally tightening up and then releasing. You can scrunch up your face, shrug your shoulders up to your ears, make fists, tighten your butt cheeks, curl your toes, and then let it all go with a big sigh.

Labels

For some of the techniques, I offer you the option of using a label. A label is a word spoken aloud or in the mind during your meditation. The label is to help facilitate mindfulness with whatever you are focusing on. If you are meditating on the body, you can say BODY silently in your mind each time you notice a sensation. If you stay with a particular sensation you can use the label every five seconds or so to help you remain focused. The label isn't a mantra—it's an acknowledgment.

The labels are totally optional. If they work for you, use them. If they don't, don't.

Feeling Overwhelmed

Sometimes, when you sit down to meditate, a lot will come up. This is especially true for beginners or anyone who is dealing with emotional challenges. Once you sit down with yourself, anything you've been holding down will rush to the surface. This is a good thing—as we all know, keeping our emotions bottled up never works for long. It's important to be brave and willing to work through this material. But it's also important to be gentle.

If you start to feel overwhelmed, it may be time to switch to a positive or restful technique. Some signs of being overwhelmed are extreme fatigue, confusion, and a fast heartbeat. You may also get angry and want to stop meditating. You might question your entire practice. Redirect your attention through some practices I'll introduce in Chapter Three, **REST AND RELAX** or **POSITIVITY BOOST**.

Remember: Be brave but gentle.

Sleepiness

It's very common to get sleepy during meditation when you first start practicing, and it makes a lot of sense. When do you close your eyes and relax your body? When you go to sleep. So it just takes a little time for your system to get used to the idea of staying awake during meditation.

If you are feeling sleepy, take a moment to lengthen your spine. This will send your mind and body the message that it's time to wake up. Or you can always open your eyes for a moment to snap out of sleepiness.

Sometimes sleepiness can be resistance. When I encounter sleepiness it usually means I'm on the edge of a big spiritual and emotional breakthrough. That can be scary, so my body will respond by telling me to go straight to bed and throw the covers over my head. Because I'm aware of that, I keep meditating.

The Quiet Mind Battle

Many people never get a meditation practice going because they can't quiet their minds. They get sick of the Quiet Mind Battle they have to wage every time they try to meditate. So, right now, before you even start, wave the white flag. Give up the fight. Cash in your chips. You are not going to win. You are a human with a brain that thinks thoughts. You don't need a quiet mind to meditate. All you need is the resolve to keep coming back to whatever you are meditating on.

When you find yourself unconsciously caught up in your thoughts, gently pick up your attention and put it back on what you are focusing on. That's it. No need to judge yourself. Getting mad at yourself for being distracted will start to infuse your meditation practice with negativity. Then you'll be less likely to meditate. Instead, celebrate that you woke up and recognized that you were mired in thoughts. This joyful and accepting attitude will strengthen your practice and your desire to meditate. Eventually thoughts will become less sticky as your relationship with your mind evolves. The mind will start to become less noisy and calmer. By giving up the battle, you'll win the war.

Meditation Prep Checklist

- ☑ Let anyone you live with know that you'll be meditating.
- ☑ Silence all electronic devices.
- ☑ Set a timer for at least ten minutes.
- ☑ Settle into your posture.
- ☑ Relax.

☑ Aim for stillness, and pause before adjusting.

☑ Don't try to quiet your mind; just refocus when you get pulled into thoughts.

The following chapter includes a whole bunch of my favorite techniques. Starting today, practice one of these meditations for at least ten minutes. You can stick with one for a week or two, or try a different one each day. As you read through the rest of the book, I'll be pointing out where a certain technique might be helpful. If you already have a meditation technique that is really working for you, great—you can use that. But it may be helpful to explore with something new too.

three
mindfulness manual: the practices

Basic Breath Awareness

This is a classic, and one that may be familiar to you even if you have never meditated. This is a version of a technique that has been taught for thousands of years, with good reason. Focusing on the breath can be very calming and grounding, and it also gets you in touch with the impermanent nature of all things. Your breath is constantly moving and changing. Each inhale is new. Each exhale is new.

For some people, focusing on the breath can bring up a sense of panic. It can feel like you are *too* aware of breathing, or that you can't get enough air. If this happens to you, try to focus on what feels good about breathing. Being very concentrated on the breath can actually be quite enjoyable. Of course, if this technique continues to make you feel anxious, don't use it. There are plenty of other options in this chapter. As you become more comfortable with meditation, you may be able to return to this technique.

For this meditation, I offer you several ways to explore the breath. Feel free to play around with all of them, moving back and forth. Or choose to stay with one. Most importantly, treat this as an adventure! The more deeply you focus on your breath, the more interesting it will become.

the practice

- Settle into your posture and relax from your head to your feet.

- Keep your attention on your body as you notice the sensations of breathing. Breathe naturally. You don't need to exaggerate your breathing.

- Place your attention on your nostrils and nasal passages. Feel the sensation of the air moving in and out. Notice how the air is warmer on the way out. Maybe you can feel your nose hairs moving as you breathe.

- Place your attention on your chest. Feel the air move in and out of your lungs. Feel your chest rise and fall with each breath. Notice all the big and little expansions and contractions as you breathe. How does it feel when your lungs are full? How does it feel when they are empty?

- Place your attention on your stomach. Feel your stomach expand as you inhale and contract as you exhale. Feel the sensation of your stomach moving against your clothing. Notice any other sensations in the stomach from breathing.

- Spread your attention out and feel the whole body as you breathe. Feel your back gently rise and fall. Feel your clothing shifting. Feel the ribs opening and closing. Notice unpleasant and pleasant sensations associated with breathing. Keep returning to your breathing body.

Rest and Relax

When I first started practicing meditation, I wanted to dive into the darkest, most painful material in my life. I was a real masochist.

I did get a lot of spiritual and emotional insight by exploring such challenging aspects, but looking back, I would have included a lot more relaxation meditation in my daily routine. I think it was somewhat traumatizing to power through so much so quickly. While meditation will improve your life in countless ways, it is strong medicine and you need gentleness as well as bravery. Today, relaxation is a very important part of my practice and my teaching. I recommend starting and ending every meditation with a period of relaxation. You can also make relaxation your whole meditation. As you strengthen your meditation skills, focusing on something that feels good is quite helpful. Your mind and body learn that meditating is enjoyable, which creates a positive feedback loop. Meditation will become something to look forward to. This positive loop can be inspired and encouraged by using relaxation as your meditation focus. REST AND RELAX helps to access deep states of rest and concentration.

REST AND RELAX can also be a powerful tool for working through difficult material. Borrowing from Peter Levine's work in Somatic Experiencing,[1] I ask students to find a resource in their bodies when working with trauma or any challenging emotions or thoughts. This means to find a place that feels okay in the body: a spot that feels relaxed, or at least more relaxed than the other areas. By focusing on that spot, you give intense emotions or thoughts a chance to cycle through, while you are safe and anchored to your resource. Even if you are not working through trauma, having a somatic resource is important for when you feel overwhelmed during meditation (or any other time).

It's very normal to start to notice everything that *isn't* relaxed when you start to practice this technique. Your attention might keep getting drawn to that knot in your shoulder or that stomachache from eating extra spicy rice for lunch. Your job here is to keep coming back to what *is* relaxed and feels good. Allow that good feeling to fill up the bandwidth of your attention. It's okay if you keep getting pulled away to discomfort (and thoughts about discomfort); just keep coming back to the relaxed area.

If you can't find a place in the body that feels relaxed, you have a few options. You can relax your body, section by section, as many times as you like. Each time, really pay attention to the sensation of the muscles in your body relaxing, even if they only relax a little bit. You can also try tightening up and releasing various muscles as I mentioned earlier. If none of that makes it possible to access a relaxed area in the body, just find a neutral place. A spot that doesn't hurt and doesn't have much sensation at all. The back of your hand, the tip of your nose, or maybe your feet. Eventually you will start to notice relaxation more easily.

As your concentration skills increase, you'll be able to focus on relaxation even if you are experiencing intense physical pain. I used this technique while I was in the hospital for some wickedly painful stomach issues. Already in immense pain, I ended up with a crazy migraine. My pain was a ten on the scale and then some. It seemed like everything hurt. As I waited for the doctors to give me some painkillers, I focused on my feet. There was no pain in my feet—they were quite relaxed. As I got some relief, I was able to notice and focus on other places in the body that were relaxed. I settled down and I stopped suffering. I was still in pain, but pain is different from suffering.

Relaxing feels good! It's okay for meditation to be something that you enjoy and get pleasure from. Feel free to put on some soothing music, wrap yourself in a soft, cozy blanket, and practice **REST AND RELAX** just to feel good.

With this technique, you have the option of using labels. Remember that labels are optional and should be used only if they help you to be more mindful. As always, you can change the label to whatever suits your fancy.

—

the practice

- Settle into your posture and relax from your head to your feet.

- After relaxing your whole body, feel for a spot that feels most relaxed. When you find an area of the body where you have the most relaxation present, focus your attention there.

- If you'd like you can use the label RELAX to acknowledge the sensation.

- Really feel the relaxation. Use your physical awareness to notice the temperature and size of the relaxed sensation. Is it spreading out or moving around?

- You can stay with this sensation or move to other relaxed sensations in the body.

- You can zoom your attention into a small area of relaxation or zoom out to cover relaxed sensations in your whole body.

- Keep coming back to what is relaxed without trying to get rid of what isn't.

- Anytime you are pulled into your thoughts, gently return to your body and the relaxed sensations you are aware of.

Pleasure Boost

The **PLEASURE BOOST** works the same way as **REST AND RELAX**. For this technique, you can follow the same directions, with the emphasis on pleasure instead of relaxation (though they are often one and the same). Try to find a source of pleasure within your body. If you'd like to use a label, try the word PLEASURE.

People often miss that there are opportunities to feel pleasure all the time. Here are just a few examples:

- Eating a delicious meal when you are really hungry
- Climbing into bed after a long day
- Peeing when you really need to
- A hot shower or bath
- That wonderful feeling after a good workout or yoga class
- Having good sex

That is a short list—there are so many more pleasurable moments throughout the day. All you need to do is start to bring your attention to them. By practicing this technique, you'll become more sensitized to instances of pleasure.

Positivity Boost

Thinking negatively and being attached to negative emotions is a habit. Like any habit, it's possible to change. The **POSITIVITY BOOST** will help you to rewire your mind to walk on the sunny side of life, without resisting or repressing the dark clouds that will inevitably arise sometimes.

In Buddhism, this type of meditation comes under the umbrella of Mettā, or loving-kindness, and is widely practiced. We send positivity to friends, lovers, family, and even enemies. Ultimately, we extend that positivity to all living beings everywhere. Science has shown that this type of meditation can decrease pain and anger, increase empathy, lower reaction to inflammation and distress, and more. It's some powerful medicine and the side effects are wonderful.

An important part of the **POSITIVITY BOOST** is smiling. This can be challenging for some people. I hear from students that it feels fake or makes them uncomfortable to smile while meditating. It doesn't matter if it feels fake—do it anyway! But don't just take it from me. You'll notice on many paintings and statues of the Buddha that he has a small smile on his face. Smiling can lead to a decrease in the stress-induced hormones that negatively affect your physical and mental health.

It's very common to be drawn to what is not positive when you first start this practice. A lot of us are in the habit of focusing on the negative. I used to do the opposite of this technique all the time. I'd even listen to music that would help me create a *Negativity* Boost! I had to work at it for a bit to create a new habit of seeing and nurturing positivity. When you find yourself being pulled into negative thoughts or painful emotions, simply return your attention to the positive material that you are creating. You don't have to try to get rid of negative images and words, just redirect your attention to the positive.

Here we will focus on offering positivity to ourselves. Later on I'll offer you some modifications to this technique that include offering positivity to others.

---

the practice

- Settle into your posture.

- Use REST AND RELAX to invite relaxation into your body. Remember, it's okay if you still have some tension in your body. This is an invitation to relax, not a battle.

- Focus your attention on what feels good in your body. You can focus on your whole body, or on a small part of it. Perhaps the muscles in your back feel particularly strong today.

- Now begin to smile. Your mind may be saying, "I don't want to smile," or, "This is fake." Don't worry about that. Smile anyway.

- Feel the sensation of your smile. Notice how it feels in your face, throat, and chest.

- Focus on whatever sensations feel best in the body and continue to smile.

- When you are ready, begin to bring some positive images to mind.

- These images can be anything that is unconditionally positive for you.

- Here are some examples that have worked for me over the years:

  Puppies and kittens.

  My nephew opening a present that he is really excited about.

  The arrivals gate at the airport. People embracing with joy.

  My own face smiling. Golden light.

- Use your imagination to create images that work for you. Move toward images that provide a positive and pleasant reaction in the body. Simply create and re-create the images.

- Now, begin to create positive words in your mind.

- Again, use your imagination to find the words that feel the best to think.

- Some examples:

   Prayers or affirmations that you like. Lyrics to a song.

   A single word that is positive for you. A sound that is positive for you.

- Directing the following phrases to yourself can be incredibly powerful:

   I love you unconditionally.

   I accept you unconditionally. You are safe.

   You are loving and lovable.

- As you focus on the positive images, words, and positive sensations, you are creating a positive loop in your mind and body. Continue to encourage and nurture this experience for the remainder of your sit.

Basic Body Awareness

Meditation introduced me to my body. Like many people, I lived from the neck up, always caught in my thoughts. When I started meditating on body sensations, a whole new world opened up for me. I felt alive in a way I had never experienced. I became aware of subtle sensations I had never noticed, and started to feel more comfortable in my skin. I also began taking better care of my body, treating it as a friend. You are with your body for your whole life and it's very important to get to know it. Your body can give you a lot of useful information if you give it your full attention.

Sometimes in my classes I'll ask everyone to share what they are feeling in their bodies. I ask them to stick to sensations, and avoid any stories. It can be almost like learning a new language. The pull to share thoughts instead of sensations is strong, but it gets easier with practice. It's amazing to discover feelings we were never aware of. We all have human bodies. Meditating on the body helps us to know ourselves and each other better.

It can feel weird and even painful to put attention on the body at first. Be patient with yourself as you practice being with your body. Over time you'll become comfortable and very skilled with using your physical awareness.

The mind can get quite loud as you attempt to take the emphasis off of what you are thinking and put it on what you are feeling. Don't try to quiet your mind if this happens. Instead just keep bringing your attention back to your body.

As you feel various sensations you may start to see images of your body. Do your best to stay with the feelings, rather than getting lost in the images. You want to feel your body with your body. The same way you can feel a textured surface like carpet or tree bark, feel the sensations in your body. Get really curious about all the elements of the sensations.

All of the techniques we have covered so far involve focusing on the body. **BASIC BODY AWARENESS** is an invitation to explore more of the sensations that might be arising. You can always come back to the sensations of breathing or relaxation.

If it's helpful for you, use the label BODY to acknowledge any sensations that you are aware of.

the practice

- Settle into your posture and relax from your head to your toes.

- Keep your attention on your body and begin to explore any sensations you are aware of.

- When you notice a sensation, give it your full attention. Soak it in. Spend a little time with it before moving on to another sensation. If it vanishes, explore your body to find another one to feel.

- Don't forget about your head and face. There are many interesting sensations in the mouth, around the eyes, in the cheeks.

- Try your best to let go of a sensation as being "good" or "bad" and just feel it as a sensation.

- Feel the size and shape of the sensations. Feel all around the edges and into the center of the sensations.

- Notice the particular qualities of each sensation. Does it feel solid or is it moving? Do you notice vibration or undulation? Can you feel a wave within the sensation? Is it expanding or contracting, or maybe doing both?

- Do not try to get rid of or hold onto a sensation. Greet every sensation with acceptance and curiosity.

- Try zooming your attention into the tiny details of a sensation.

- Now, try zooming out to cover sensations in your whole body.

- Keep returning to the body, no matter how interesting and important your thoughts seem.

- Finish your meditation with some relaxation as outlined earlier in REST AND RELAX.

Focus on Emotions

This is a technique for meditating on emotional sensations in the body. It can help to get you out of the story in your mind and into the actual physical experience, allowing you to "sit with your feelings" with acceptance and curiosity.

If I were to ask you how you feel today, what would you say? Nine times out of ten, people respond with a story about what's going on in their life. This is how most people relate to their emotions: as a list of thoughts. But emotions are actually sensations in the body, which is quite different.

If you are feeling sad, your throat might feel tight, or you might feel pressure in the chest. If you are crazy over the moon in love, you might feel an expansive warmth in the chest. If your boss took credit for an idea of yours, your skin might feel hot with anger. **FOCUS ON EMOTIONS** is a technique to help you get in touch with your emotional sensations, separate from thoughts.

Why would you want to do this? Let's say you are going through a breakup, and the decision to end the relationship was not mutual. You are suffering. If you were practiced in meditating on emotions, you could begin to separate the sensations from the thoughts. By doing this the experience becomes less overwhelming: It is just some sensations, albeit uncomfortable ones, and some words and images in your mind. You realize that if you are observing your emotions, you are not your emotions. You are able to accept the experience and allow it to move through you. Suffering ceases, and while you may still be in pain, you are no longer in agony. You are better equipped to take care of yourself through the transition.

Grasping at pleasurable experiences and resisting painful experiences leads to suffering. Being mindful about emotions allows you to greet all experiences with equanimity. Generally, the good things get better and the bad are not so bad. **FOCUS ON EMOTIONS** works the same way as **BASIC BODY AWARENESS**, except you'll only be paying attention to sensations that have an emotional flavor. For a lot of people, emotional sensations show up in the face, throat, chest, and stomach. You may notice them in other areas too. If you are unsure if a sensation is emotional, just take a guess. If you are not aware of any emotions in the body, just use **BASIC BODY AWARENESS** instead. Be open to the possibility that some emotion may arise, and attend to it if it does. You have the option of using the label EMOTION for this technique. The label can be particularly useful when working with challenging emotions.

—

the practice

You can follow the same directions as **BASIC BODY AWARENESS**, but focus specifically on emotional sensations. Remember that you are not trying to create emotions, you are just noticing what is there. You don't need to know what the emotion is or why it's there. Just noticing that it seems emotional and focusing on it is all you need to do. Remember not to resist or grasp at sensations. Be with whatever arises, offering the sensations acceptance.

If you are having trouble locating emotional sensations, here is an exercise to help sensitize yourself to them.

- Settle into your posture.

- Bring up in your mind a moment in the last week or month when you felt sad, angry, or embarrassed. Recall this situation and any other people who were involved.

- Notice what happens in your body as you think about this.

- What do you feel in your face, throat, chest, and stomach?

- Explore the sensations for a few minutes. Greet the sensations with acceptance and curiosity.

- Now let that go completely.

- Bring up in your mind a moment in the last week or month that you felt happy, peaceful, or proud. Recall the situation and any other people who were involved.

- Notice what happens in your body as you think about this.

- What do you feel in your face, throat, chest, and stomach?

- Explore the sensations for a few minutes. Greet the sensations with acceptance and curiosity.

- Feel free to now move into the PLEASURE BOOST.

Focus on Mind

This technique is what got me to start meditating daily. Like many people, I was convinced that I had to quiet my mind in order to meditate. I would get all bent out of shape about the nonstop chatter in my mind, and I would usually just give up. When I was introduced to meditating on the mind, all that changed. The mental talk and images became something to meditate on, and suddenly meditation was something I could do.

If we are attached to our thoughts, it leads to suffering. We think we are our thoughts, and we believe what we think. Thoughts that tell us we are not good enough, not attractive enough, or not rich enough rule our lives and dictate our moods. But it's possible to be liberated, and this technique is a great path to that liberation. To practice FOCUS ON MIND you will put your attention on your thoughts. Not the content of your thoughts, but rather the *activity* of your thoughts. It doesn't matter if the words or images seem really important or really mundane. During your meditation you'll greet any and all thoughts with acceptance, just listening to them come and go. Get interested in the way the words and images bubble up and then vanish. Don't try to create, hold on to, or push thoughts away; just observe and explore with as much acceptance and curiosity as you can. Eventually you'll be able to listen to the mental talk as if it were someone else speaking and watch the images without becoming attached.

The first insight people usually have with this technique is that they realize how much is going on in the mind all the time. Not only is the mind constantly babbling, it's usually blurting out pretty negative content. That can be a painful realization, but it's a big step toward getting freedom from the tyranny of the mind. I was shocked by how noisy and nasty my mind was when I started to investigate. I have found that over time, through my meditation practice, my mind has settled down quite a bit. When negative thoughts do arise, I'm able to notice them in the moment and choose not to believe them.

You have the option of using the labels TALK (for mental talk) and IMAGE (for mental image). For many people, using the label TALK is not helpful because a label is mental talk, but try it out and find out how it works for you.

—

the practice

- Settle into your posture and relax from your head to your toes.

- Place your attention in the area where mental talk arises for you. For most people it happens in the head, but it might be somewhere else for you.

- If there is mental talk arising, listen to it. Not to the content, but to the activity of it: the arising and passing away of the words. It could be a narration on your meditation, a list of things you're going to do later, or the replaying of a conversation. It might be a song, or even just tones. Observe any mental talk with acceptance and curiosity.

- Notice the volume, pitch, and pace of the mental talk. Notice the beginnings and endings of thoughts.

- If you find yourself pulled into the thoughts in an unmindful way, come back to listening with more detachment. It doesn't matter what your mind is saying—it's all just mental talk.

- If there is no mental talk, just be with the quiet until some arises.

- Now let that go and bring your attention to the area when mental images arise. For most people it happens around the eyes, but it could be somewhere else for you.

- If images are available, look at them. Be less interested in the story of the images and instead explore the activity: the coming and going of images.

- The images may be of your body, or the room you are in. They might seem to be on a screen or all around you. They could be thin and wispy, and you may not be sure what they are. It doesn't matter what they are; just keep observing with acceptance and curiosity.

- If there are no images, gaze into the space of no image.

- Keep your eyes relaxed. There's no need to strain; allow the images or empty space to come to you.

- Now you can begin to observe both mental talk and images. You may be able to notice both arising at the same time, or you may want to move back and forth between the two. It also may be the case that only one is available. If so, focus on that one.

- Finish your meditation with REST AND RELAX or the POSITIVITY BOOST.

Focus on Self

This technique changed my life. It's my go-to meditation and one of my favorites to teach. FOCUS ON SELF is an insight technique that combines FOCUS ON MIND and FOCUS ON EMOTIONS. This meditation allows you to observe how thoughts and emotions influence each other, and ultimately create a sense of self. This sense of self can be deconstructed through meditation, showing you that you are not as solid as you might think.

All experiences, pleasurable or not, occur to us through both thought and emotion. Take this moment, for example. Take in this idea of all of your experiences, your very sense of self, being made of nothing more than thought and emotion. What is your reaction to this concept? Does it excite you or scare you? Now, notice what your reaction is made of. It's made of words and images in your mind and emotional sensations in your body.

This is actually really good news. When you start to realize that you are more than your thoughts and emotions, you begin to have a choice in how you want to move in the world.

To practice FOCUS ON SELF, simply combine FOCUS ON MIND and FOCUS ON EMOTION. Allow your attention to free float between all three (self, mind, and emotion). You can use the labels EMO-TION, TALK, and IMAGE if that is helpful for you. When you are focused on one of these three, *know* that you are focused on it. When you find experience tangled up and yourself taking it all personally, come back to witnessing with curious acceptance. Don't forget to reconstruct yourself using the POSITIVITY BOOST at the end of your meditation.

Meditation in Action

In essence, this whole book is about meditation in action. You will be learning to bring your meditation practice into sex, but you can also bring it into all other aspects of life. Here are a few examples of ways you can practice.

Walking Meditation

Walking meditation is a big part of Zen practice. Find a safe area to walk, either in your home or outside. Choose to either walk back and forth in a limited area or have an extended walk. Start by bringing your attention to the sensation of your feet on the ground. Feel one foot lift as another touches down. You may wish to stay with that or expand your attention to other sensations associated with walking. As you become more practiced, you can practice any of the techniques discussed earlier in this chapter while walking.

Workout Meditation

Put your headphones aside and try bringing your meditation practice with you to the gym. Focus on the muscles that are working hard. Feel the movement of your body. Some people find it helpful to focus on good feelings in the body during a workout using the **PLEASURE BOOST**.

Dishwashing Meditation

Dirty dishes can become a fantastic meditation. Put your attention on your hands. Feel the warmth of the soapy water, the weight of the dishes, and the cool rush of water as you rinse.

Stream of Consciousness Writing

Free writing is another kind of meditation. We are making the unconscious conscious when we write in this way. Get a new journal or notebook to use while you read this book. There will be many times when I suggest you do some stream of consciousness writing after an exercise. When you are writing in this way, don't worry about how it sounds or if you are spelling a word correctly. Instead, just let it spill out onto the page. Let the words surprise you. Don't censor yourself.

You now have an arsenal of tools and techniques for making meditation a daily habit. If you practice even just one of the included techniques daily for the next few months, you will notice the benefits.

Remember, things will come up when you sit in meditation. It's helpful to have a teacher and a community to support you. If you have a partner, meditate with them and talk about your experience afterward. There are even online communities that can help you along the way. For some, seeking out the support of a therapist can be the right way to go. These days there are many therapists who incorporate mindfulness into their sessions.

Every time you sit down to meditate will be different. Sometimes you'll be bored, sore, and tangled up with thought. The time will move like molasses. Other times you'll be overcome with a blissful experience. Ten minutes will feel like one minute. Don't get attached to the "good" meditations. It's all a good meditation, even when it seems like nothing much is happening. Sometimes you'll end up getting more out of a humdrum sit than you will out of a sensational one. Don't judge your practice; just do it.

These techniques are meant to wake you up to yourself and the present moment. They also lead to many insights of an emotional, intellectual, sexual, and spiritual nature. Yes, meditation is great at lowering stress and anxiety, helping you sleep, giving you more concentration at work or school, and improving sex. But what it was originally intended for is waking up. Waking up to suffering and the end of suffering. Waking up to the beauty, mystery, and awe in every pebble and every drop of dew. Waking up to what you really are. So, as you practice, you will find yourself becoming more awake. For some, awakening is a smooth ride, and for others it is fraught with many bumps and roadblocks. Sometimes things fall apart before they come together—that may be the case for you. It was for me.

four
feelin' it

Even during my early encounters in which I didn't always value the quality of my sexual experiences, my sex life has always been very important to me. I've seen sex as a creative way to connect with myself and other people. You might say it's been my hobby, or my extreme sport. For a big chunk of my sexually active years, though, I was selling myself (and my partners) short. I was not in touch with my body. I couldn't feel the subtle vibrations after an orgasm ends, or the warmth that spreads across my inner thighs and stomach when I become aroused, or the tingle in my chest when I get kissed exactly the way I like.

When I started practicing meditation, I didn't set out to have better sex. In fact, I didn't actually know what I was missing at that time. I set out to process years of painful emotional buildup and hopefully to grow spiritually. I didn't know that by sitting quietly each day and exploring the sensations in my body, I would start having mind-blowing sex. It makes sense, though. The more I got to know my body, the more it could offer me.

I go to silent meditation retreats at least once a year. It's a time to put my regular life on pause and dive deep into my practice. On the first night of a recent retreat, the teacher, a Buddhist nun, said, "Go to sleep tonight for the first time. It's the first time every time. It's brand new. It's the only time." This is how I try to live my life, from my head hitting the pillow to giving head. Each time is brand new; each time is the only time.

When you encounter your sexuality as something mysterious and unique, your fixed ideas and emotional and mental blocks can begin to melt away. Sex becomes a beautiful dance. Rigidity gives way to fluidity. The default setting of your lovemaking is replaced by endless possibility, surprise, and awe.

How do we begin to bring this freshness into our sexual expression? The first place to start is where you are right now. In your body.

The Impermanent Body

Before we take one breath of air outside of our mother's womb, we already have a body. Until the last breath we take before death, we have a body. Our bodies experience birth, pain, pleasure, emotion, illness, old age, and ultimately death. Our bodies are always with us.

Mindfulness is about being right here, right now. And when you are moving toward mindful sex, it's of the utmost importance to be grounded in your body. It is in the body where the sex is happening, after all! Even so, we spend a lot of time resisting our bodies. There are many reasons people don't want to be grounded in their bodies. Chronic pain, sexual trauma, and stress can all make the body seem like an enemy. For me, the body was not a safe place to reside. I had a lot of physical pain from a young age. Back issues, chronic headaches, digestive problems, and more. I was accustomed to finding ways to get out of my body to relieve pain, whether it was emotional or purely physical. There was anger, sadness, and trauma stored up inside my skin. Being embodied made me feel afraid and stressed-out. I couldn't do yoga because it was too uncomfortable to hang out with my body for that long. I used to have murderous fantasies when someone put their mat too close to mine. There was a lot of anger piled up inside of me. The body is also an ever-present sign that illness, old age, and death are a part of life. You are going to get wrinkles and gray hair; you will experience illness; and eventually you'll drop dead. The body is a big, flashing neon sign of a reminder that everything is impermanent. It can be difficult to look at that sign and accept it for what it is.

But when we ignore illness, old age, and death, we resist a huge part of life. We are basically pretending that the story won't end the way we all know it will. This resistance and denial causes us a lot of unnecessary suffering. Whenever there is resistance, we are taking a chunk out of our potential to experience the fullness of life and of sex.

You might think you can avoid pain by staying out of the body. But when you actually feel the pain and accept it, your relationship with it changes. When you get grounded in your body, you come to realize that pain is just another sensation to be experienced. You'll also find that it changes. It gets stronger and weaker, disappears completely, flares back up, and disappears again. Pain may continue to ebb and flow, but you will no longer be suffering so much. The level of discomfort will become the right size. Your body offers you a chance to experience impermanence with every ache and pain.

You need to be in your body to really feel all the good stuff, too. Your body has so many ways to create pleasure and it all feels better when you really *feel* it. Think about how enjoyable a hot bath is when you are cold or have sore muscles. How about getting a massage from a skilled bodyworker? Or the feeling of being in love? Those pleasurable feelings can all be heightened with mindfulness.

When you are in your body, you get the full experience of pleasure, not a watered-down one.

You would think that everyone would want to be in their bodies during sex. It feels good, right? But many people are having disembodied sex. I used to be one of them. I felt the broad strokes (like climax), but all the subtle sensation was ignored. Even our orgasms are greatly limited when we aren't mindful with the body. There is so much more to be felt when we bring mindfulness to our bodies during sex.

Learning to be present with pleasure in the body can also help us not to be so attached to it. Attachment to fundamentally impermanent things is a recipe for disappointment. Acceptance is the antidote for attachment, and being fully present with an experience will lead to acceptance. I also find that letting go of my grasp on pleasure makes it all the more pleasurable. I like to breathe, relax, and let go. It's hard to really enjoy sex or anything else if you are holding on for fear of it ending. Here's the thing: It will end. Everything does. When we greet and bid adieu to pleasure with acceptance and curiosity, when we hang on loosely, it is free to delight us in a whole new way.

Learning New Tricks

I often hear from people about "that one amazing time" they had, and how they just want to get back to that. Some go so far as to use the memory of a good lay to get off every time they have sex. There is certainly nothing wrong with recalling especially satisfying sessions. I've laughed with partners about how a really hot time can keep the fires burning for weeks between us. Just the mention of it is all the foreplay we need! But overly relying on memories to be able to have pleasure during sex is limiting and disconnects us from our partner. We are just replaying the past like a movie in our minds instead of actively engaging with the present moment. Fantasy absolutely has a place in mindful sex, but we don't want it to be our only option.

I know letting go of what works for you, what gets you off, can be hard to do. But I promise you it will be worth it. You can also come back to your old tricks from time to time, or maybe expand upon them. Being more grounded in your body will only make these tricks better anyway. Nurturing a relationship with your body will give you a new blueprint for pleasure. You will wonder how you ever had sex without the emphasis on embodiment. That has certainly been my experience.

When teaching others to have what I call *embodied sex*, I like to start with masturbation. When I first began wanting to bring mindfulness into sex, I didn't have anyone to practice with, so I did it by myself. It was a wonderful way to get to know my body and my capacity for pleasure. Even if you have a partner who is game, it might be helpful to get in touch with your sexuality on your own first. Sometimes it can be a bit too confronting to jump into embodied sex with someone else, and mindful masturbation is a gentle way to begin the journey.

I'm going to suggest something that may feel unfair and bring up resistance for some. For this exercise, please don't use sex toys, porn, or fantasy. This isn't going to be about getting off, it's about getting into the body. This is a meditation to help you stay with your body as you experience sexual sensations.

Create a safe, cozy, soft space to practice this in. Your bed, a couch, or even the floor with pillows and blankets will all work. You may also wish to have your favorite lubricant handy.

the practice

- Set a timer for ten or fifteen minutes and lie on your back in a comfortable position.

- Take a moment to relax from your head to your toes.

- Start by touching your face. Run your fingers down your cheeks and jawline. Trace your lips with your fingertips. Use BASIC BODY AWARENESS to tune into the sensations.

- Focus on the pleasure, as you learned to do in the PLEASURE BOOST, but stay open to all sensations, including the subtle and even the uncomfortable.

- As soon as you find you have been pulled into thought, come back to sensation. Move your hands over your neck and collarbones.

- If you have breasts, take some time to explore them. Keep feeling the sensations, without judging them.

- Some of the sensations may be very pleasurable and some may not. Just keep noticing how your body feels.

- Touch your stomach and sides.

- Really feel every touch, returning to the body when you start getting tangled up with the mind.

- Now start to ever so gently brush your fingers over your genitals. Don't jump right into doing what you always do, instead softly explore.

- Let go of the outcome and get curious about the sensations. You may wish to use some lubricant at this time.

- Touch the most sensitive spots, the least sensitive spots, and everything in between. Let this be a brand new experience. Recognize this as the first time.

- If you feel the strong urge to hurry up and climax, relax and don't pursue that urge. There is no goal to this other than learning to be with your body.

- Treat your genitals like you are touching them for the first time. Get to know them.

- If you have testicles, you can explore them as well. Try squeezing, pulling, and touching very gently. Press the area between your testicles and anus.

- If you have a vagina, try putting a few fingers inside, getting to know that area too. The clit is actually quite long. Feel the outer portion, on top of the hood and under it, and the inner portion. Notice how it swells and throbs.

- Keep coming back to the sensations in your body.

- Continue to explore your genitals with a fresh and curious attitude until the timer goes off.

When the timer goes off, congratulate yourself. You have taken a big first step to more connected and mindful sex! If you are feeling turned on and want to bring yourself to climax after the exercise, go for it. But before you do, take a moment to notice how this experience made you feel. What did you like about it? What did you hate? Did you find that your mind became noisier at certain points? Were there any new sensations that you never noticed before? This would be a good time to grab your journal and do a little stream of consciousness writing about how you feel.

If you do decide to go back to masturbating after this period of contemplation, do your best to stay with the sensations—even if you use the old standard technique, including toys and whatever else tickles your fancy, to come. Try to stay with the body as you orgasm, rather than checking out to get off.

To be clear, this isn't how I masturbate every time, or how I think you should. This is a special exercise to help you connect with your body. I'm simply inviting you to give yourself more options. When you are first learning to have embodied sex, putting aside distractions is helpful, but that doesn't mean that what turns you on is wrong. There's no need to judge yourself or become too rigid—just be willing to give something new a try. You may find that by temporarily closing one door, three more open.

Loving the Skin You're In

Another reason embodied sex can be a little scary is that many people don't like their bodies. Being in the body during sex is a reminder that the shape, size, or appearance of your body is not quite right. This isn't true, of course. You are perfect just as you are in this moment. But I know it can be hard to believe that, and the world around us doesn't always help.

While there has been a movement against body-shaming in recent years, the message is still pretty clear: You are not thin enough, or you are too thin; your muscles are too small, or they are too big; your breasts are too saggy, or they are too small; your skin is too dark, your skin is too light; your penis is not the right shape; your belly is too round—*you are not good enough as you are.* The pressure to be considered attractive is pounded into us everywhere we go. Commercials, films, and television show us what we *should* look like, and that content seeps into our consciousness. We starve, inject, and brutalize our bodies in hopes of meeting an imaginary standard of beauty. We reject this beautiful vessel that is here to serve us. This high level of self-hatred and denial in our culture really hurts our chances of having embodied sex.

I'm not saying we shouldn't eat healthy, get good exercise, and make an effort to look nice. Heck, I love the way yoga makes my butt look. I eat so clean it's embarrassing, I like wearing makeup and heels

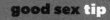
good sex tip

A word about using lubrication: I'm a big fan. Even if you create plenty of fluids, it can aid in exploration and help you to focus on sensation. With some of the exercises in this book, you may or may not be turned on, so lubrication can be helpful. People with penises can also get a lot more enjoyment by using lubrication for masturbation. Make sure to use water- or silicone-based lubricant if you are using a condom or dental dam. Oil-based lubricant can weaken the barrier of your protection.

and I may have tried a little Botox. But we need to nurture a loving and accepting attitude toward our bodies. From a place of self-love, we can make choices that are right for our own unique body. When we love ourselves, it becomes natural to take care of our bodies.

Here's a self-love exercise that often makes people grimace and groan. If you think it's dumb, pointless, and embarrassing, then you should definitely do it. It can be done with your eyes closed or while looking in the mirror. This will help to rewire your mind to see yourself as you truly are—perfect and totally lovable.

the practice

- Close your eyes or look into your own eyes in a mirror.
- Allow your eyes, jaw, and shoulders to relax. Say these phrases out loud to yourself:

    I love you unconditionally.

    I accept you unconditionally.

    You are beautiful and lovable just as you are.

    Repeat the phrases several times.

That's it! You survived. It's kind of funny how much resistance there can sometimes be to offering yourself love. It's okay to treat yourself with love and kindness. It's also okay to fake it 'til you make it. If you are wired to put yourself down, it can take time to create new neural pathways. But you can do it if you consistently offer yourself kind and loving words daily.

Self-love and acceptance are paramount for embodied sex. Learning to love and accept yourself is an ongoing process, and one helps the other. As you get more mindful with yourself, you'll get more mindful with sex, and vice versa. I know that for some people the preceding exercise is not easy. Be gentle and patient with yourself. This is not a race or another thing to "get right." I've been working on self-love and acceptance for years and I haven't graduated yet! Learning to love ourselves, and by extension others, is our life work. There is no finish line, as far as I can tell.

A Whole New World

Learning to be embodied with someone else is the beginning of a whole new kind of sex. I love hearing from clients after their first embodied sexual experience. They say things like: *I never knew I could feel so much*; *I felt so connected to my partner*; *My orgasm went on forever*; *I had no idea it could be like this*. People also find that the benefits spill over into all aspects of life. Work feels easier, creativity gets freed up, there's more patience for the kids or other family members, the world is brighter and more beautiful, and a sense of relaxation and ease replaces stress and tension. Discovering embodied sex is its own kind of spiritual awakening.

I also get another kind of report. For some, embodied sex is incredibly confronting. Being in the body during sex can be very challenging. Sometimes, just the grief for the years of disembodied sex can be overwhelming. As always, patience, self-love, and acceptance is the antidote for this kind of experience. We can't get around this material—we need to go through it.

Before I started down the path to wellness and spiritual evolution, I avoided partners who encouraged me to be embodied during sex. I thought they were too emotional, too sensitive, and too needy. Imagine thinking someone is needy for wanting you to actually be in your body during sex. But that's how my mind worked at the time. When I first began having embodied sex it was like waking up from a deep, dark sleep. My eyes opened to a world that I could hardly comprehend.

Reading about embodied sex is great, but doing it is better. Before we plunge into sex, let's try it with a hug. Mindful hugging is a fantastic way to test out our new embodiment skills. It's also something you can practice with a friend in a platonic way if you are single or don't have a willing partner.

This practice will introduce you to your body and help you to build the concentration to stay with it. As you become more comfortable residing in the body, you can start to bring that new awareness into your sex life. This means staying with the sensations of your body while engaging with someone else. It can be tempting to go back to thinking about sex instead of feeling sex. As you develop your concentration skills, you'll get better and better at being present to the body sensations of making love.

—

the practice

- Agree on an amount of time for the hug and set a timer. A minute is a good place to start.

- With your clothes on, standing up, face your partner. Step forward until you are close enough to comfortably wrap your arms around each other. Stand up straight and feel grounded.

- Relax your body. Hug.

- Use BASIC BREATH AWARENESS to get in touch with the body. Feel your own breath moving in and out.

- After you feel present with the breath, start to expand your attention outward using BASIC BODY AWARENESS to notice the sensations of hugging.

- How does your face feel? What about your stomach? Feel your arms and your legs. Notice the feeling of your body touching your partner's. Feel your partner's heartbeat, breath, the warmth of their body, and the pressure of their arms around you.

- You may want to close your eyes to help you focus on the sensation of hugging. Take your time with this, even if it feels silly.

- Notice and really feel all the sensations that arise.

- Sometimes this exercise can bring up challenging emotions and lots of thoughts. Try your best to stay with the good sensations of hugging. Scan through your body and notice if you are tightening up anywhere. Release that tension.

- When you are done hugging, take a few minutes to talk about the experience. Share in detail what it felt like for you and listen to your partner's experience.

If you are doing this exercise with your partner, a lot can come up. For example, who usually ends a hug first? And who is usually left wanting more? What does that say about other areas of the relationship and how does that play out in your sex life? This exercise will begin to open up those questions, so please be patient and gentle with each other and yourselves. Having mindful sex includes being mindful with each other's lovely and tender hearts.

The first few times I practiced this exercise, I wanted to jump out of my skin. It was so uncomfortable to allow myself to soften and relax in my partner's arms. My heart would start beating fast and my breath would become shallow. Over time, I became more comfortable relaxing while embracing. It just takes practice and lots of self-love and mindful soothing. Now Mindful Hugging is one of my favorite things to do.

Putting Your Practice into Action

I was always a very serious person, even as a kid. I was called a "little grown-up." I remember winning an award in my early twenties. I was so serious in my acceptance speech that I came off as cold and ungrateful. I now know that I acted that way because I felt too vulnerable being expressive and joyous.

Sex was always one place that I could stop being so serious, but only to a point. I still wanted to do it "right," and I wanted my partners to do it right. Whatever I deemed to be right, that is. There wasn't a lot of room for playfulness and humor. Those were both luxuries that my checked-out self could not afford. As I integrated my mindfulness practice into sex, something marvelous happened. I started to play and have fun. The seriousness began to melt away as I softened into a less severe version of me. I like to say that I am getting younger and younger the older I get. There is a childlike wonder and joy that blossoms when you don't take things so seriously.

When you are ready to bring your new body awareness into sex, remember to take it easy. There is no need to get super serious and bogged down with technique. If you go into it with the goal of "getting it right," it will feel more like doing your taxes than having sex. There is no "right way" of having mindful sex. Allow some playfulness and lightness to enter the scene. Have fun!

Just like with mindful masturbation, I would suggest that you forego sex toys, fantasy, porn, or any other default turn-on when you start practicing embodied sex. You can always add it back in, but for now, start with getting grounded in your body. It may also be helpful to take orgasm off the table in the early days of embodied sex. We can get so focused on getting off that our body awareness becomes very limited. You might choose to have intentionally embodied sex for a set amount of time, treating it like a meditation. If, after that period of time, you want to pull out the vibrator collection and focus on the Big O, go for it. You may find that eventually embodied sex becomes the new normal, and toys and fantasy are just an occasional cherry on top.

Ideally, this is something you can share with your partner, but that isn't always the case. If your partner is not interested in all of this mindful sex stuff, you can still try it out for yourself. If you find yourself feeling resentful that your partner doesn't want to explore mindful sex with you, take a moment to turn the spotlight back on yourself. Where in the relationship are you resistant? Are there parts of the relationship that you don't bring mindfulness to? How can you be more present with your partner? Of course, sometimes your partner's resistance to mindful sex may be showing you that you have outgrown the relationship. Before making that decision, address all the ways you could stand to evolve. Take your time and do your best.

The only thing you really need to do to have embodied sex is *to be in the body*. Focus on your body before you start having sex. What does it feel like when you know you are about to get intimate? Explore the tingles and shivers of anticipation. Feel the earthy heaviness of your body, alive with longing. Notice how your genitals begin to throb or become warm with blood. Whenever you find yourself pulled into thoughts, bring your attention right back to your amazing body. Stay with your body as you kiss and touch. Stay with your body when you take safe sex measures. Sometimes when the condom, glove, or dental dam comes out we can check out a bit. Instead, let that be a part of the experience.

Stay with the body when giving or receiving oral sex. While I am a big proponent of open-eyed sex, it might be helpful to close your eyes during oral sex to focus on the sensations. As you become more comfortable residing in the body during sex, open your eyes and enjoy the view!

Whatever sex means to you, whether it involves penetration or not, stay with your body while you do it. If you and your partner are taking this adventure together, you can support each other. One way of doing this is to name the sensations you are feeling. By saying what you are experiencing out loud, you'll help you and your partner stay focused on your bodies. It can seem kind of silly, but try it out. Use descriptive words and get specific about where in your body you are experiencing the sensation (*I'm feeling a deep throb in my clit. I'm feeling a sweet shiver in my legs. I'm feeling a tingling warmth in my chest.*) As always, there's no wrong way to do this, so give yourself space to explore. If talking takes you out of your body too much, you may want to save sensation naming for later.

Get deeply interested in all the elements of sensation. Notice tingles, throbs, waves, heat or coldness, vibration, contraction, expansion, and undulation.

Direct your physical awareness to sensations of pleasure, without resisting any uncomfortable feelings. You may realize that you like something you never noticed before or that you don't like something that you thought you did. If you discover that something your partner is doing doesn't feel good, tell them. Express yourself in a kind and loving way. Focusing on sensations of pleasure is a great way to become more mindful during sex. All you need to do is really feel the pleasure of sex. You can focus your attention in just one spot, move from sensation to sensation, or expand your awareness over your whole body. Deeply tune into what pleasure actually feels like. Get present with each throb, each rush of heat, and each tingle. Focus on the sensations of touching your partner. Experience the movement of your hands on their skin, the feeling of their hair in your hands, the wetness of the sweat on their body. If you love the way your partner tastes and smells, take that in as completely as possible. You can start to experience not only your own pleasure more fully, but also the pleasure of making your partner feel good more fully. There have been times when it seems like I can actually feel what my partner is feeling.

Once you are really feeling the sensations of sex, start noticing the movement and change in the sensations. There is the movement of your breath and heartbeat. There is the movement of your partner's body against yours. Soak in this flow of changing sensations. During oral sex is a good time to practice this concentration. Focus on the flow of pleasure in your body and on the movement of your partner's mouth. Merge those sensations together in your awareness for a really connected experience with your lover. There is an endless flow of sensations in your and your partner's bodies.

Feeling your way into that flow is a way to enhance your pleasure and your intimacy with your partner.

Anytime you get pulled into thought or a sense of grasping, just come back to the pleasant sensations of sex. Remember: Orgasm is not the goal or the end of the experience. You don't need to worry about coming too soon or taking too long. There is lots of pleasure to be had and to offer regardless of when or if you orgasm. Anchor yourself in your body and go along for the ride.

Use the tools of **BASIC BODY AWARENESS** to help you stay with the sensations that feel good during sex. You will find that there is much more sensitivity in the body. It may be overwhelming at first, so go slow and check in with yourself and your partner along the way. If you need to go back to mindful hugging to ground yourself, that's totally fine. Let it be fun! Taking yourself too seriously can make it harder to be present and really feel what's going on.

Bring these new skills into every area of lovemaking. That includes flirting, foreplay, kissing, and everything else. Watching your partner take off their silk tank top, or recognizing the scent of their cologne when they come into the room can create all kinds of sexy sensations. There are so many opportunities to enjoy the experience of your body while being intimate with your partner. If you don't have someone to practice with, try it on your own. Use your body awareness skills to explore the experience of self-pleasure.

Talking and writing about the experience of embodied sex is a wonderful thing to do for yourself. This gives you a chance to integrate the mind with what has physically occurred. Consider doing a little check-in with your partner after sex to discuss your experiences. Think of this as a chance to express any discoveries or feelings that arose during the session. If you want to share something that didn't go quite the way you wanted, be gentle. This is about collaboration, not critique.

Remember to be patient. It's easy to get frustrated in the beginning of a meditation practice and that is true of learning to bring mindfulness into sex too. If the experience isn't what you had hoped at first, you are not "doing it wrong." You are learning a whole new way of relating to yourself and your partner. This requires lots and lots of love and kindness. As you continue to practice embodied sex, it will feel more natural and easeful. I always want to race to the finish line when I'm learning something new, so I know how that feels. Over the years I've gotten much better at being on the journey without asking, "Are we there yet?" over and over. Slow down and enjoy the ride.

This and This

An important insight on the spiritual path is that you are not your body. Your body is a part of what you are, but you are not reducible to it. As you sit in meditation and observe the plethora of sensations that arise and pass, it becomes clear that you are not those sensations. If you can witness them, you must be something else.

However, this is only one side of the coin. On the other side, you are deeply connected and one with your body and every sensation in it, no matter how small. Tricky, huh? Well, you'll have to get used to this nondual way of looking at things. If you keep your meditation practice you won't have to get used to it, you'll just come to know it.

One way of thinking about enlightenment is this: knowing deeply that there is no self, but having the ability to manifest a self as needed. Part of that self that arises is your body. You have been gifted, at birth, with this fabulous concoction of cells, organs, bones, skin, limbs, and features.

Learning to let go of attachment to the body while at the same time caring for and *enjoying* the body is a worthy endeavor. When you no longer identify with your body as you, you have a freedom to more fully sink into the body and connect sexually. If you keep meditating, you'll start to get a sneaking suspicion that you are not what you thought you were. You will see that you are so much more than a body. Follow that thread and explore it for yourself. But as you gain this insight, remember that it's only one part of the spiritual path. Embodiment is equally powerful and enlightening. Everything you need for awakening—and for the best sex of your life—is right there in your body.

five

open-eyed love

I can't tell you how many times I have heard people say things like this about their partners: *I really love my partner. We have so much in common. They are so kind and supportive. They remembered when I mentioned how much I liked that coat and gave it to me for my birthday. Their family doesn't drive me crazy! We could win an award for Best Spooning of All Time. They listen to me, really listen to me. They are an extraordinary pool player. They are the best co-parent I could have ever hoped for . . . but our sex life sucks.*

My first question is: *Do you talk about it?* People often say yes, but when I dig a little deeper, it's clear that communication is not really happening. Brushing it off with a joke doesn't count. Only bringing it up when you're drunk doesn't count either. Neither does talking your friend or therapist's ear off about it. The conversation needs to happen in an honest and present way with your partner. This means sitting down next to each other and honestly discussing your sexual needs and desires.

From what I've seen in my work, many people are not having honest communication about sex with their partners because they can't do it with themselves. That can make it rather hard to open up and express deep sexual desires, fantasies, and preferences. Learning to listen to your body and communicate your needs takes practice and patience, but it's a worthy endeavor and an important part of good sex.

We all have an inner voice or intuition that very clearly states what is true for us. You know what I'm talking about. It's that part of you that tells you not to go on a second date with someone, or when it's time to leave a job. This voice will also tell you what really turns you on, which sexual position you love, and which you don't. That voice will reveal your most secret fantasies and deepest longings. You just need to listen and then be willing to speak your truth.

Not all of your inner voice will come in the form of thought. Sometimes your voice will be somatic, expressed through your body in the form of emotional sensations. That's where **FOCUS ON EMOTIONS** can be particularly insightful. Getting to know your emotional body is key in learning to communicate with yourself. Tracking and observing emotional sensations in your daily meditation practice will make it easier to be aware of your emotional landscape at all times, including during sex. Your body will give you incredibly clear messages. Your job is to listen to what it's saying and then communicate what you feel.

When I started to truly be in communication with my emotional body, it was like having a whole new sense. I could feel my feelings, not just think about them. After years stuck in my mind, it was so liberating to have more space to experience myself. It was also irritating sometimes. My mind would be telling me to do one thing and my body would be pulling the brakes! It took some time for me to trust this new relationship with my body. There were lots of times I went with what my brain wanted to do and ended up regretting it. I found myself in jobs and friendships that my body couldn't stand, but my mind thought was okay. After enough suffering, I became willing to let my body lead the way. I continued to use **FOCUS ON EMOTIONS** to deconstruct my emotions and to find more equanimity with the challenging bits. Now, I trust my body implicitly. I need look no further than the sensations I feel to make a decision these days. This kind of self-communication is part of what made mindful sex a reality for me.

The Body Knows

The best place to start communicating with your body is in your daily meditation practice. By using **FOCUS ON EMOTIONS** regularly, you'll begin to get to know your emotional self. You will start to know where and how you experience sadness, joy, embarrassment, lust, and all the rest of your rainbow of emotions. You will realize that you can experience conflicting emotions at the same time. We are amazing and complex creatures, but when we are fixated on one emotion, we forget that. It is revolutionary to develop the ability to notice and allow irritation to exist but focus on joy instead. While mindfulness is never about getting rid of your emotions, it does give you the power to choose what you want to pay attention to.

You'll need to learn to tell the emotional sensations apart from the non-emotional ones. In general, emotional sensations can often be detected in the face, throat, chest, and stomach, though you may experience them elsewhere. An itch, a headache, or back pain wouldn't necessarily be considered emotional, but they could create an emotional reaction in the body. You are the ultimate judge on what is deemed an emotional sensation, and it's okay to guess! Is it nervousness in your stomach or just indigestion? You get to decide. The more you work with this technique the easier it will be to tell emotional from non-emotional. There can also be overlap between the two.

As you become more trained at observing and exploring emotional sensations it will be easier to understand what your body is communicating. It's no different from learning a new language. It just takes practice. You will find that you can identify these emotions as you are walking about, on your way to work, or in the grocery store. You'll start being able to practice meditation in action.

I used to get so mad if someone cut in front of me in a line. I felt as if the line-cutter had set out to personally offend and disrespect me. I would get so angry and bent out of shape that it would affect my day for hours to come.

Then, one day, after I had a little meditation in action under my belt, it happened. Someone cut in front of me at a smoothie shop. But this time something was different. I could feel the anger rising in my body, in the form of a tightening in my chest and a heat on my skin. I could hear the thoughts about how rude that person was. These were separate strands of experience. I was able to observe them separately so that they didn't become tangled and put me in a bad mood for the rest of the day. I stayed with this mental and emotional phenomena, exploring it and getting curious. Before I knew it, the emotional sensations and thoughts had vanished. I wasn't angry anymore. I even smiled at the person who had cut in line as he walked out with his bright pink smoothie.

We all have our pet peeves. If you practice noticing emotional sensations during one of these episodes, the first thing you'll be aware of is fear. Maybe a cold, tight feeling in your chest and a racing heartbeat. You will be able to process that as it occurs, noticing the sensations with acceptance. If you're a black belt in mindfulness, you may not even get to the anger part. The anger is most likely trying to hide the fear. But we can't be ninjas all the time, so maybe you get angry. Anger is also made up of sensations in your body. If you don't get caught in the story of the anger, you can feel the sensations grow and then fall away. The fear and anger don't stay in your body because you have fully allowed the emotions to move through.

Communicating with your body can improve your life. There is a huge amount of freedom that comes from getting to know your emotional body. No longer needing to resist the unpleasant feelings or grasp at the pleasant ones, you'll be free to delight in the beautiful flow of sensations. I have found that even the challenging parts of experience have taken on a kind of beauty these days. That doesn't mean I'm never sad or angry, but I have a new clarity and relationship with the emotional process.

This new clarity will of course come into play in your sex life. It will mean knowing what you want less of *and* what you want a whole lot more of. Your body will give you all the info you need, from which condoms it likes best to which positions cause discomfort. If you are willing to listen, your body will show you pleasures you never thought possible. But you'll need to take that communication to the next step for the full benefits. You'll need to speak the truths your body is telling you out loud to your partner.

Let's Talk about Sex, Baby

I understand the anxiety about asking for what you want. It was so hard for me to express my sexual wants and needs in the past that I could only do it when I was drunk. When I gave up drinking I had to start voicing my desires while stone cold sober. At first it felt terrible and I could barely get the words out. I was worried of being judged or rejected, or just sounding silly. It was hard for me to be open about anything, let alone sex. The intimacy of sharing openly and allowing another person to see me was a foreign concept. It made me feel weak and dangerously vulnerable. Growing up in a dysfunctional home had taught me to hold my emotions in and only count on myself. It took time and practice to trust that it was safe to show my inner self to someone else.

FOCUS ON SELF is a great tool when learning to talk about sex. This technique allows you to notice any shyness, fear, or discomfort in the body and mind, without judging your experience. Offering yourself this space and acceptance will gently encourage you to share with your partner what turns you on and what doesn't. Here is a special exercise to help you become more comfortable talking about sex:

the practice

- Sit comfortably and relax from your head to your toes.

- Take a moment to bring to mind what you'd like to say to your partner about your sex life.

- Imagine yourself having the conversation. Notice what happens in your body when you think about having that conversation. Gently rest your attention on those sensations. Just feel them without trying to change them in any way.

- Notice if any images or words arise in your mind in reaction to imagining the conversation. Don't try to stop or change them, just notice what comes up. Be accepting and curious about whatever happens in your body and mind.

- After you have mindfully attended to what came up, take a moment to again imagine talking to your partner.

- This time, imagine the conversation going really well. Imagine that you are both relaxed, open, and loving. See your partner hearing you and see yourself feeling heard and understood.

- If a thought or emotion contradicts this positive experience you are creating, gently bring your attention back to the image of a loving interaction.

This exercise gives you a chance to explore some of what might come up for you as you begin to communicate about sex. It also helps you to imagine a positive outcome. This isn't about getting attached to a particular expectation. It's more about priming you to be in a positive frame of mind. Focusing on the positive will feel good and influence the way you communicate for the better. If you have big emotional and mental reactions to this exercise, you may want to use it to practice until you are ready to talk with your partner.

Stream of consciousness writing is also a great way to become more comfortable communicating about sex. Try writing down all your desires and fantasies. Don't censor yourself at all. Be willing to write down whatever comes to mind even if it's something you wouldn't actually want to *do*. It's okay to have fantasies that you don't actually want to live out. Get it all out; then repeat the practice again a few days later. Allow this to be a fun and creative experiment. You can burn or shred the pages when you are done, or you may decide to turn some of this writing into a sexy letter for your partner.

Letting your thoughts come out on the page will give you some relief from the nasty tyrant in your mind. The story that says it's not appropriate to talk about sex. The fearful mental loops about being rejected or misunderstood. The voice that says you'll get it wrong, that you are not good enough. We can become so congested with fearful and self-centered thinking that it becomes impossible to communicate. Observing thoughts in meditation and letting them empty out on the page will help you to detach from them. Once you have a clearer perspective there is more room to explore your sexuality with curiosity and ease. Then, sharing that part of you with someone else becomes more possible.

What Do You Want?

A good next step is to talk about sex when you are not having sex. That can take some of the pressure off of you and your partner. It will be best if you start the talk when you can both be relaxed and present. Choose a time when neither of you has time constraints. Don't replay the conversation over and over in your mind, trying to find the perfect way of stating your feelings. If you find you are doing this, practice some stream of consciousness writing. Get it all out on the page and then let go of being perfect. If you are still feeling nervous or stuck in the mind, take a moment to relax from your head to your toes before initiating the discussion.

Sit comfortably next to your partner, rather than across from them. Start slow and stay in touch with how your body feels as you talk. Notice if that tyrant in the brain starts spewing nonsense. Don't try to turn off the thoughts, just set them aside and come back to connecting with your partner. It's okay to tell your partner that it's difficult for you. Consider speaking some of the sensations you are feeling out loud. Just saying, *Wow. My stomach just got really tight*, can help ease the discomfort and increase the intimacy. Sharing how you feel when you talk about sex is talking about sex! It's also okay to laugh and allow for fun. Don't take yourself too seriously.

If you are on the receiving end and your partner shares a desire with you, never judge or criticize them. If what they are asking for is out of your comfort zone, be gentle and offer another option.

To be able to hold space for your partner, you'll need to be able to hold space for yourself. It can be hard to hear that your partner wants to make a change in your sex life. It can feel like you've done something wrong. In fact, it's the opposite. You've done something very right if you are in a relationship that allows for this level of communication. There can be some fear, even if you are all for trying what your partner has proposed. That's okay and perfectly normal. Change, even for the better, can be uncomfortable. Notice the thoughts and emotions that come up for you, and pause before responding. That mindful pause can be the difference between a warm loving exchange and very hurt feelings.

Collaboration Is Sexy

Becoming more comfortable asking for what you want during sex doesn't mean you'll always get what you want. You might think your girlfriend would look super hot in a naughty schoolgirl outfit, but she may think, *No way in hell.* Some fantasies may need to be put aside. The great thing is that there are endless possibilities. Let your sexuality be creative and flexible. You and your partner have the wonderful task of collaborating to create the best sex for both of you. It's a work of living art that you can continue to develop over time. Collaboration is something that has taken me a while to become comfortable with. I was very much a gal who took care of herself and didn't expect help. In fact, if someone wanted to help with or add to something I was doing I became protective and defensive. It was just one of the many ways that I was checked out and shut down. As I peeled back the layers of defensiveness using my meditation practice, collaboration became more possible. One of the first places I saw the change was in my sex life. I could open myself up to my partner during sex in ways that I might not be able to on something like a creative project, for example. Mindful collaboration with sex has since given way to an ability to collaborate in all kinds of ways.

Part of sexual communication and collaboration is expressing what you don't want. If a certain position doesn't feel good for you, let your partner know. It's important to be kind and open when letting someone know that what they are doing isn't working for you.

Framing your needs in a collaborative way will keep you and your partner on the same team working toward mutual pleasure. Stay in touch with your emotions while having sex, and let your body tell you what it wants. It's okay to stop in the middle of a sex act if it isn't feeling good to you. Don't ever feel that you have to "finish what you started." Mindful sex means taking care of yourself and never ignoring what is true for you. Consent is fluid and a *yes, keep going* can sometimes turn into a *no, please stop*.

Right Speech

There is nothing like blaming, criticism, and dishonesty to remove any chance of good sex. If you are harboring resentment or anger toward your partner, it will come out even if you think you've got the lid on it. It will be in the tone of your voice when you say, *Oh, is it my turn to load the dishwasher?* It will be in your body language when you are silently driving to a dinner party together. It will be in the roll of your eyes when they tell that same old joke to a group of friends. If you are not speaking with kindness and truth, communication becomes a messy and painful affair.

Before my meditation practice, I had many romantic relationships in which I was not practicing Right Speech—not communicating with compassion. While I didn't intend to outright lie, I would often bend the truth or leave out key details. I did lots of little things, like using a dismissive or condescending tone, or ever so slightly poking my partner in an emotional tender spot. Rather than encourage and inspire my partners, I belittled and competed with them. Looking back, it's very clear to me why I behaved this way. I was dishonest and unkind to myself, which made it impossible to treat my partners with love, honesty, and respect. I was also afraid of the intimacy that comes with kindness and trust. I felt that I needed to protect myself from getting screwed over or rejected. My wiring, when it came to communication, was faulty.

If you grew up in a home where good communication skills were not being practiced, like I did, you may be familiar with this faulty wiring. The bar was set very low for me when it came to mindful, loving communication. The fact that I wasn't telling big lies or screaming at my partners made me think I was succeeding at having a functional relationship. In reality, I was missing out on the kind of relationship we all deserve. A relationship built on kindness and honesty is the only kind of relationship in which good sex can happen. This is the case even with a friend with benefits, or a one-night stand. Healthy communication is required for a fulfilling sexual interaction of any kind.

Right Speech starts with how we talk to ourselves. Until I learned to speak kindly and truthfully to myself, I couldn't do it with anyone else. One of the early insights that many of my students express is discovering how nasty they are to themselves in their minds. It's as if the voices in our minds are hell-bent on convincing us we are not attractive enough, not smart enough, not rich enough, not good enough. I have never come across someone who hasn't at some point been able to relate to this experience. Our minds can be real bullies. So how do we become aware of our negative self-talk, and learn to talk to ourselves in a more caring way? This is where **FOCUS ON MIND** comes in.

good sex tip

Maybe you want to be spanked or tied up, but telling someone to dominate you doesn't feel very submissive. This is where talking about it beforehand is helpful. You can ask your partner to surprise you when you are least expecting it. Mindful communication beforehand about boundaries (including establishing a safe word) is essential when experimenting in this way.

If you want to create a new relationship with your thoughts and the way they manifest in your communication with your romantic partners, start by getting to know your mind. Choose an amount of time (I'd suggest ninety days) to practice **FOCUS ON MIND**. Every day spend at least ten minutes working with this technique. **FOCUS ON MIND** gives you the option of paying attention to both visual and auditory thinking. For this period of time, try just observing the mental talk. You'll find that the words and images often arise together, but do your best to separate them and limit your attention to only the words. At first it may feel challenging. It can be a bit of a brain twister. Stick with it and soon you'll be able to listen to your auditory thinking as if it were someone else speaking. This is a huge insight into the nature of the mind. It points right to something all spiritual teachers will agree with. You are not your mind.

That insight makes it easy to stop believing, overvaluing, and acting on everything you think. You then have the freedom to choose what thoughts to give merit and what thoughts to set aside. Notice, this isn't about "quieting" the mind. Instead, you are empowering yourself to get the most out of what your mind has to offer. Your mind is a tool—a very powerful tool. When you start to learn to use your mind instead of being used *by* your mind, wonderful things can happen. One of these wonderful things is that you no longer get attached to the mean stuff your mind has to say. This detachment from negative thinking allows you to put Right Speech into action.

If You Don't Have Anything Nice to Say

Right Speech will facilitate good interactions in all of our relationships. When we set the intention to speak with truth and kindness at work, with our partners, with our children, with our extended family, and even with strangers, we are creating opportunities for a deeper and more fulfilling connection. Right Speech also absolutely lends itself to better sex. I don't know about you, but if someone speaks unkindly to me or lies to me, my sexual attraction to them takes a nosedive. On the other hand, I find kindness and honesty to be a big turn-on.

Learning to share your desires with a partner is much easier if you are both practicing Right Speech. When you are naked and in the midst of having sex, you can feel pretty vulnerable. An unmindful word can be devastating. As you ask for what you want and express what you don't, let kindness be your foundation.

There are kind, mindful ways of communicating even your most hurt feelings. I like the saying, *If it's important, it's not urgent.* I've found it to be true, except in a few specific situations. If you are in an abusive relationship, it is important and urgent to get out. Other than that, there is always time to slow down and sit with what you are feeling. That can make it much easier to communicate your feelings in a caring, productive way.

If you have any resentments regarding your sex life, take the time to clean your emotional house. During sex is not the time to air your grievances, even if they are carefully hidden inside of other words. That sort of subtext can be felt and will not open the door for fun and constructive dialog. I suggest uncovering your resentments and understanding what your part is in the situation. If you're feeling upset with your partner for not having energy for sex at the end of the day, first look at yourself. Take a look at areas you could stand to improve. Do you greet your partner with a loving attitude at the end of the day, taking time to connect in nonsexual ways? Do you offer other options to sex like a bubble bath together or trading massages? Do you come to bed in the evening already tense, expecting rejection, or from a place of openness and love?

Whatever the issue you have with your partner, there are most likely ways that you are falling short too. An effective way to find your part is to get your resentments down on paper. Write it all out, even if it feels petty or not enlightened enough. Once you've poured it all out on paper, take some time to consider and write down in what ways you've contributed to the problem. Sometimes it can be quite obvious, and sometimes it takes a bit of soul-searching. It can be helpful to talk it out with a therapist, coach, or good friend who will take an unbiased view. When you know your part, you can get to work on being the change! When you are free from resentment or blaming, talking about sex will be much easier.

Eyes Wide Open

Talking is not the only way to communicate during sex. Our eyes can express more than our words in many instances. If you are like a lot of people, this idea is completely foreign, if not horrifying. I found this out when I started teaching and writing about mindful sex. I've had many people tell me that they have never looked into their partner's eyes while having sex. A lot of folks talk about the awkward eye contact that sometimes happens by mistake, and how they quickly look away and squeeze their eyes shut. That doesn't make for open, connected, and mindful sex.

Some people feel they will "lose their concentration" if they open their eyes, as if sex is a math test. You'll find that you become much more deeply concentrated when you pay more attention to the other person. In fact, you may find yourself in a very special kind of concentrated state. This type of concentration feels amazing and incredibly easy once you access it. The same way an athlete can drop into "the

84

flow" during a competition, you can get in "the flow" while making love. Many people spend their entire spiritual career focused only on this meditative state of profound stillness and concentration. When you are "in flow" your mind becomes fully immersed and absorbed in your object of focus. In the case of open-eyed sex, the object of attention would be your partner's eyes and body.

For some, it seems too lovey-dovey to make eye contact. They feel it's something reserved for "making love" and they want to fuck. Actually, eye contact during fucking is incredibly hot and adds to the raw intensity. But don't take my word for it. Try it for yourself. I dare you.

Other people say they enjoy eye contact during sex but can't keep it when they are going into orgasm. They say, again, that they need to concentrate. As you bring more mindfulness into your sex you'll find that this tight, buckled-down kind of concentration is not required to get off. It's just a habit and it can be changed. The reward for taking the time to let go of this old model of orgasmic concentration is connecting with your partner while you climax. Your wild eyes and open mouth will blow their mind.

Being Seen

The main reason I see for the absence of eye contact during sex and orgasm is that it is scary to be seen. Often, the other reasons are just masking this fear. I get it. It *is* scary to let others see you.

When I was fourteen, I went to a Quaker Youth camp. It was a week of self-empowerment, community building, and creative exploration. One day, I went to an acting workshop thinking it would be fun and help me with my budding acting career. The first exercise was to walk across the room twice in front of the group. The first time you were to walk as you presented yourself to the world. The second time you were supposed to walk the way you *really* felt. My first walk was with a puffed up chest, and an armor of confidence and cool. As I began the second walk my body became hunched and my face became heavy with sadness. Suddenly, I collapsed on the floor, sobbing. I had let this group of people see how I really felt, and it hurt. It made me aware of how I really felt deep inside. This experience didn't wake me up at the time, but it stuck with me. Over the years, as I healed from my childhood trauma and learned to love myself, I began to want to be seen by others. Today, I seek that kind of intimacy in all my interactions with the people in my life.

Being literally seen during sex can feel confronting and bring up uncomfortable emotions. Don't let this keep you from exploring open-eyed sex. Learning to soothe and comfort yourself will help you to tolerate these feelings. One way you can do this is to open your eyes for ten seconds or so, feel the fear or insecurity arise, and then close your eyes and just focus on the good feelings of sex. You can keep adding a little more time to the open eyed periods, resting in the sensations when you become overwhelmed. You may wish to think a few self-loving thoughts, too. If you feel comfortable doing so, I'd suggest telling your partner what you are working with so they can support, inspire, and encourage you. That's where your verbal communication skills come back in.

FOCUS ON SELF can be a big help when learning to have open-eyed sex. You can deconstruct the discomfort into thoughts and body emotions to make it less powerful. Using this practice daily will help you to access it easily during sex. As you bring mindful attention to the uneasy thoughts and feelings that come when you open your eyes, you'll find you are less attached to them and more focused on being in the moment with your partner.

Being able to make eye-contact during sex increases intimacy and pleasure. It also gives you the chance to have some incredible communication. By actually seeing your partner's face, you'll know if you're moving your hips just right, or if you are thrusting just a little too hard. Often words won't be necessary to let you know if you should speed up or slow down. A twinkle in your partner's eyes will inform you to pull out some favorite toys. While it's important to learn to ask for what you want by speaking, it sure is nice to be this connected with someone. It can feel like you're reading each other's minds.

Oh Say Can You See

Another obvious feature of open-eyed sex is that you can see what is happening. Your body and your partner's body moving and merging. The curves, muscles, and drips of sweat. Open-eyed sex is one way that guys can get incredibly turned on. This can be true for women as well, but studies have shown that men are more sexually aroused by visual stimuli.[1] Guys, try out a little visual meditation on your partner's body. You will probably find it quite easy to concentrate.

I'm not suggesting that you always keep your eyes open during sex or for every orgasm. Sometimes it's really nice to close your eyes and just enjoy the sensations. Nor do you need to lock eyes and never blink or look away like intimacy robots. But it's valuable to have the option to open your eyes, see your partner, and let your partner see you. Flexibility and fluidity are important tenets of good sex. Even if you choose to have your eyes closed for most of your sex session, give yourself the choice. Having variety available is sexy.

If you're not quite ready to have open-eyed sex, try eye-to-eye meditation with your partner first. This is a beautiful way to build intimacy and to get more accustomed to extended eye contact. Just like with mindful hugging, this doesn't have to be done with someone you are sexual with. So if you don't have a partner, ask a close friend to do it with you.

Eye to Eye Meditation

The first time my partner and I tried this technique, we set the timer for thirty minutes and hunkered down for some extended eye contact. We were both already very comfortable looking into each other's eyes and we fell into a deep meditation right away. As I focused on his eyes, I began to feel waves of pleasure through my body. Anytime a thought arose, his eyes easily brought me back. I found that I was becoming totally absorbed, my concentration strong and unwavering. Being concentrated in this way is one of the most pleasurable experiences I have had. Usually it only happens on retreat or when I'm meditating for several hours a day, but just looking into my partner's eyes gave me access to this wonderful stillness and focus. I no longer could tell my body from his. Our inherent oneness was revealing itself. At some point we both realized that our meditation had been going on for a long time. I looked down at my phone and discovered that the timer had never gone off. We had been gazing into each other's eyes for almost an hour and a half.

—

the practice

- Make sure the room is lit well enough to see each other easily. Set a timer and sit across from your partner. Not too close and not too far apart. You want to be able to comfortably focus on their eyes.

- Take a moment to relax from your head to your toes while looking into your partner's eyes. You may find it is easier to focus on just one eye at a time.

- Now simply look into your partner's eyes, in a relaxed way, without straining.

- Allow your partner's features to blur as their eyes become sharper and clearer in your vision.

- As you notice sensations arise in your body, allow that to be a part of your experience, while still focusing on your partner's eyes.

- Whenever you find yourself being pulled into thinking, come back to the eyes. If your eyes get tired you can try defocusing them for a moment or closing them briefly. It's okay to blink! Just don't close your eyes and retreat inward—you and your partner are supporting this practice together.

- Allow any emotional sensations to arise and pass.

- As sensations flow through you, you may start to feel more and more connected to your partner. Let the boundary between you and your partner become thinner and thinner as you gaze into their eyes.

Aftercare is very important with this technique. Looking into someone's eyes for even ten minutes is outrageously intimate. All kinds of emotions can surface. I suggest taking a few minutes to cuddle and then talk about the experience. You may both want to do some stream of consciousness writing as well. You may also feel like you have excess energy running through your body. Use it to work on a creative project, or have some wild sex!

good sex tip

Something I get asked about a lot Is how to feel more comfortable "talking dirty." Many people feel really shy and embarrassed about whispering sweet nothings or telling naughty tales to their partners. This makes sense— it is a kind of performance and requires you to access your creative juices. Like learning to perform as an actor or musician, talking dirty takes practice. It's okay to "fail" miserably and laugh at the funny things that came out of your mouth. It might take some time to find your stride, but keep at it and you'll become a pro. It's also okay if talking dirty isn't your thing. It's not really mine, but I love for my partners to do it. Explore and don't let fear of "getting it wrong" stand in your way.

Sex without Separation

Learning to communicate with your partner is necessary for a rich, exciting, and hot sex life. It's also another path to spiritual awakening. The awakening to your own truth through listening to what your body has to tell you. The awakening of trust and connection with your partner. The awakening of love and compassion as you get to know you partner more deeply. As you connect more and more during sex, you begin to sink into a whole new level of awakened communication.

There is a kind of communication that can occur during sex, which requires no words. Every slight movement, every breath, and every look speaks on a level deeper than language. This type of connection is something we all long for, even if we don't yet know it. The first time you experience this kind of communication, a spark lights up in the depths of your being. A remembering. This profound communion with your partner points to an insight that you've always had. There is no separation, no duality. As you move and breathe with your partner you are shown that you are connected with everyone and everything, without exception.

crazy mindful love

Romantic relationships are one of the most life-affirming and exciting experiences that a human can have. They also make you grow. David Schnarch, PhD, author of *The Passionate Marriage*, calls marriage (or a committed relationship) a *People-Growing Process*.[1] Part of the way this process does its job is by triggering the heck out of you and uncovering the unconscious material that had been neatly tucked away while you were single. A good relationship should chew you up and spit you out as a wiser, kinder, and more awake person.

I see romantic relationships as one of the great teachers and healers that we have. They can bring you right back to your humanity and heal your deepest emotional wounds with a sometimes gentle, sometimes fierce grace. Every partner I've had has taught me something valuable and ultimately lead to deeper healing. In that way, I find that every lover and every sexual encounter thrusts me into a new layer of awakening.

When you see your romantic partners as part of your psychospiritual growth, you begin to value them more. Even the moments of conflict become an opportunity to awaken more fully, love more deeply, and heal more completely.

There are many opportunities to get the maximum juice out of a relationship, even if your current partner doesn't turn out to be your lifelong partner. By being mindful at the very beginning, you'll give yourself a chance to make the most of the beautiful and messy thing that romantic love is.

Love Drugs

She was a sexy soft butch. From the moment I saw her—surrounded by admirers in a badly lit bar—I was hooked. After a few weeks of her kisses and cunnilingus, I was obsessed and crazy over her. All I could think about was her and our possible future together. Would we travel through Europe, making love in Italian hostels and smoking fine hash in Amsterdam? Would she write me poetry and love beach camping as much as I do? I was writing a romantic novel in my head.

The high I felt when she called or when I was with her was exquisite. The lows, when our dates ended or when she didn't answer my calls, were extremely painful. After spending a weekend together, mostly in bed, I was spun out like I'd been doing blow for days. I needed more. My heart was pounding out of my chest and my mind was going a million miles a minute. I couldn't eat, couldn't sleep, couldn't concentrate on anything. I was high on Love Drugs.

The excruciating pleasure and pain of the first flush of love is like nothing else (well, some studies have shown that it's remarkably similar to cocaine addiction).[2] Until I was a meditation practitioner, I was all too willing to completely lose my mind during that time. I loved to completely check out of my life by getting lost in the insanity.

You know how it goes. You are on the freeway, madly texting the object of your desire, risking your life and the lives of others to send just one more witty response. You are missing work because you haven't been able to practice basic self-care, and you've come down with a Love Flu. You are checking your phone fifteen times an hour, looking back over the old texts if a new one hasn't come in yet. You think you see them everywhere, and each time your heart starts speeding and your skin gets hot. They don't text back and it feels like someone has pulled your plug and emptied you out. Your lover is all you can think about.

It's one thing to enjoy this experience. It's another thing to use it as a way to check out. As you wake up more and more through your spiritual life, you don't want to go back to sleep in your daily life. Your spiritual life and your daily life become one and the same. Staying awake means being willing to change the way you relate to everything, including the extreme highs and lows of romantic infatuation.

What if, instead of losing our minds over a new relationship, we stayed awake during this process? What if we opened ourselves up to a whole new way of experiencing new infatuations? Love Drugs create a great opportunity to work with craving and attachment in a very hands-on way.

Getting Sober

The first time I worked mindfully with the agony and ecstasy of attraction, it took all of my skills. I found it incredibly challenging to simply observe the thoughts and emotions that were arising. Building a new set of tools takes time and practice. I had been getting high off of Love Drugs since I was a gangly, wild-haired eleven-year-old, and those grooves in my brain were deep. At that age, I had things going on in my life that were too painful to be present for. The massive crush on the boy with freckles who lived in my neighborhood or the excitement of skinny-dipping with my pretty best friend gave me a reprieve from the chaos at home. Infatuation with a love interest was a useful way for me to avoid uncomfortable emotions for many years.

As I started to wake up, my meditation practice asked me to give that up. But I started to get the sense that letting go of my attachment to Love Drugs would be hard, and I didn't want to do it.

My writing, teaching, and personal practice is all about letting go and waking up. I deeply believe that this is what I am here to do. This letting go and waking up allows me to truly connect with others and live authentically. And sometimes it sucks. Sometimes spiritually evolving means losing things you really don't want to lose.

In my case, seeing through the Love Drugs meant letting go of the part of me that could still get high off of them. It meant coming out of hiding a little bit more and giving up the escape that an intense crush can bring.

Eventually I asked myself: Why would I stay unconscious around this? It may feel like losing something, but I'm only losing a false reality. So, I'm not actually losing anything at all. Part of having a spiritual awakening in our sex lives is about being willing to let go of who we think we are and what we think we know. It's about giving up the option of checking out or escaping through sex and romance. If love looks a lot like addiction, then it's no surprise when a person uses it a lot like an addiction to escape unpleasant realities. And it was time for me to end that.

Then something remarkable happened. Once I stopped being able to consistently get high off the love/sex experience, it began to seem crude, disruptive, and even silly. It's important to be open to all of our experience, so I tried not to resist that either. I laughed out loud when I felt that chemical rush through my body. It was so predictable. The less I was pulled into the intensity, the more I could just witness the rise and fall of sensations and thoughts. They stopped being "me," and I stopped needing to do anything about them.

That doesn't mean that I didn't continue to have fun texting, flirting with, and fucking my new love interest. Rather, I was able to let go even more into the experience because I was not grasping so much. This brought a deeper connection with the other person and allowed me to interact from a place beyond the stories my mind generates. I saw the other person as a unique and spectacular human, not just as a way to get high and check out.

This shift changes things. If you are someone who gets a big "fix" from romantic and sexual intrigue, be ready to lose that. It's not going to be the same once you see through the chemical, emotional, and psychological response. You won't be able to get high in that way anymore. It will take time to discover what your sexuality looks like without the attachment to the highs and lows of Love Drugs.

Kicking the Habit

Here are some quick and dirty tips for taking the first few steps to letting go of Love Drugs:

- Pause before you send that text to your crush. Practice **FOCUS ON EMOTIONS**. Notice what it feels like in your chest, stomach, and lower regions. After you send the text, pause again. Notice what it feels like. Just be with those sensations for a moment. While you wait for a response, especially if it doesn't come as quickly as you would like, pause again. Pay attention to your body. Feel your body with your body.

- Pay attention to what happens in your mind and body when you get a text or phone call from your honey, potential honey, or "if only" honey. Get curious about the rush of sensations, both the pleasurable and uncomfortable ones.

- When you notice your mind looping back on itself while thinking about someone, observe your thoughts. Use **FOCUS ON MIND**. Recognize that you are not the thoughts; you are observing the thoughts. Stop taking the thoughts so personally and just listen to the sound of the words, and see the images arise and pass.

- Once you can observe your thoughts, notice all the space around the experience. The pulsing of sexual excitement, adoration, or craving is only one small part of what is happening. Your attention can become very narrow, and the thoughts and emotions around this person will be all that you see. But awareness is much, much bigger. If you rest in awareness, you will cease to become your grasping. Instead, it will just be one of the many waves in an endless sea.

Being attached to the Love Drugs moving through our bodies, or the stories in our minds, creates a separation. When we no longer hold on to what we want or brace ourselves for disappointment, we get to be right here right now. There's not much that's hotter than that.

good sex tip

There is nothing wrong with having sex on the first date, but what if you waited? Let the sexual energy build over a few weeks before going all the way. Get to know your desire and enjoy the waves of pleasure that come with wanting.

Working through Challenges

Conflict is unavoidable in romantic relationships. If you are conflict-avoidant, as I have been at times, you'll need to take a look at that. Intimate relationships ask us to roll up our sleeves and get in the mud.

If you find that you are faced with tons of conflict within the first few months of a relationship, you may want to reassess. Ideally, those beginning days of a relationship are a time for fun and exploration. If there are already a bunch of red flags, perhaps you've bitten off more than you can chew. Or maybe you are just taking it too seriously. Relax and enjoy the ride. There will be plenty of time to dig into the challenges of merging your life with another human.

As your relationship matures, it will be time to put a different kind of work in. Here are a few key things that I find incredibly helpful when navigating relationships, especially in the first few tumultuous years.

The Magnifying Glass and the Mirror

Eventually, the Love Drugs will wear off and you will be left, sober, with each other. This is when all the cute, neurotic things about your partner start to annoy you. The way they eat, the humming they do while driving, the throat-clearing, the way they leave the toilet paper sitting on top of the toilet instead of putting it on the roll, how fast (or slow) they tell a story about their day, their "lucky underwear" that have holes in them but cannot be thrown out. All of this becomes downright irritating, and you know that the honeymoon is over. Or is it? If experienced mindfully, this stage of a relationship can actually be fertile ground for personal growth and deepening intimacy with your partner.

When we are feeling uncomfortable about something in ourselves, it's common to start noticing what we don't like about our partners. The moment I get annoyed with some trivial thing that my partner does, I can be sure that there is something going on with me that I don't want to look at. It's easy to avoid or resist our own shortcomings or unconscious material when we are picking apart our partner. This is when you need to put away the magnifying glass and take a look in the mirror instead. In this way, the things that annoy you turn into opportunities to grow. As soon as I take a look at myself and figure out what I'm trying to avoid, my irritation almost always vanishes.

If you are ultra-focused on what other people or institutions are doing wrong, you may miss what you could stand to improve in yourself. There may be times that you are sure you're right and *they* are wrong, but don't be so sure. Judgmental black-and-white thinking, even about things that seem obviously wrong, will keep you safely separated from your own shadow side. Mindfulness asks us to pause when feeling agitated, angry, or defensive. In that pause, you have a chance to look within and get down to the heart of the matter.

What Is My Part?

When your partner is doing the thing that most bothers you, it can be hard to stop on a dime and look at your part. But that is exactly what is needed in those moments. It takes humility and skill to be willing to see our part, especially when we are feeling triggered and defensive. We can gain that skill through practice, just like we gain any other skill.

You can practice in the moment, which can be challenging at first, and you can also practice in writing and meditation. If you make this exercise a regular practice, your relationship will benefit greatly.

—

the practice

- Write down the resentment or hurt feelings you are experiencing. Include all the details. Get it all down.

- Sit down with a notebook and pen close by.

- Take a moment to relax from your head to your toes.

- Now, bring to mind a conflict you have with your partner or anyone else. Allow the thoughts and emotions to arise without resistance.

- Ask the question: How is this affecting me?

- Without grasping for an answer, allow an answer to arise. It's okay if the answer is, *I don't know.*

- Sit with this for a few minutes and, if necessary, ask the question again.

- Now ask the question: What is my part in this situation?

- Without grasping for an answer, allow an answer to arise. It's okay if the answer is, *I don't know*.

- Sit with this for a few minutes and, if necessary, ask the question again.

- Now do some stream of consciousness writing about whatever came up in the meditation.

- You may find that you want to move back and forth from writing to meditation a few times.

It is possible that your part could be simply showing up for mistreatment. Then you'll need to continue to explore and find out why you think you deserve to be mistreated. It could be that you are not being so nice to yourself, and therefore finding others to replicate that. I did that for years. I treated myself terribly and then wondered why I often fell hard for people who didn't treat me very well. Once I started treating myself with love and respect, the scenery around me changed quite a bit. Work on you and nurture your self-love, and the rest will take care of itself. There is an exception to this: *If you are in a physically abusive situation, the first priority is to get somewhere safe.* Once you are out of danger, you can take a look at your part.

Loving Kindness

A powerful way to work with conflict is to send positivity to the person you are at odds with. In doing this, you begin to wire your mind toward a loving and positive attitude, rather than an angry, blaming, or annoyed one. You'll find that when you send loving kindness to others your perspective of them changes, as does the way you interact with them. This version of the POSITIVITY BOOST can be used with anyone: a boss, parent, friend, or even a politician you don't like! At first it can be hard to think kind thoughts for someone you are pissed at, but it's worth working through the resistance.

When I was in my mid-twenties, my girlfriend and I broke up after a year and a half of a super dysfunctional relationship. My feelings were deeply hurt when she immediately began dating someone I had always suspected she had a thing for. I felt so rejected and brokenhearted and all I could think about was the two of them together. Someone suggested that I try praying for them. I translated that into a kind of positive meditation for them and practiced it for three months anytime they came to mind. At first it was really hard, I couldn't even get through it, but eventually it got easier. Then I bumped into them at an event. After all those months of focusing on kind and loving thoughts about them, I actually felt good when I saw them. My mind had been trained to think positive thoughts about them. It was a smooth and painless interaction and it made me a true believer in the power of positivity.

If you are experiencing resentment toward your partner (or anyone else), try this practice daily for at least a week and/or anytime you feel resentment.

—

the practice

- Take three deep breaths, in through your nose and out through your mouth with a big exhale.

- Now say the following phrases in your mind:

  May (insert person's name) be happy. May they be healthy.

  May they live with ease.

> May they have peace, serenity, abundance, and love.
>
> May they feel comfort and happiness.
>
> May they know that they are lovable just as they are in this moment.
>
> I release this resentment toward them.

Depending on the person and situation, this can be really challenging. It's an advanced practice, but it will also advance your practice.

Water Meets Its Own Level

I used to agonize about whether I should stay in a relationship or leave. I had a lot of dysfunctional relationships, so I spent a great deal of time thinking about it. Then one day someone wise said something to me that changed my life. She said, *Water meets its own level.* We tend to partner with people who match our own psychological awareness levels. Until my own sea level changed, I'd keep finding myself with people who mistreated me.

This can be difficult to hear, and difficult to express without edging close to victim blaming, but in an abusive relationship, it's not always just the abuser who needs to work on themselves. The abusive behavior comes from some sort of unconscious fear, insecurity, or trauma. And it can be the same thing with the person who takes all of the abuse. They might have some unconscious material that makes them believe, on some level, that an abusive relationship is what they deserve.

I've been on the receiving end of abusive relationships: jealous fits, broken windows, bruises, blood, police, jail, all of it. While abuse is never an acceptable response, at that time of my life I had a huge amount of work to do on myself. I was bringing my own share of dysfunction to the table. Relationships like that allowed me to ignore myself and put all the focus on my partner and how terrible they were. This made it possible for me to be lazy about the personal work I desperately needed to do. Once I started to address what was going on with me and why I felt drawn to abusive partners, the people that came into my life changed. My water level had shifted.

If you are waffling about whether you should stay or cut and run, here's the simple truth. If you put the focus on your personal growth, one of three things will happen: (1) your partner will grow with you and you'll continue on in the relationship; (2) your partner will grow but it will be in a different direction and you'll break up; (3) or, your partner will drag their heels, not grow much at all, and you will move on easily. You will have moved to a different water level and it just won't work anymore. You no longer have to think about it—just keep working on you! Remember that you can't *make* your partner grow, or grow in the way that you want. Focus on making your own changes and let things take care of themselves.

This philosophy is not limited to romantic relationships. It goes for friends, therapists, teachers, and work too. If I put the emphasis on my own emotional, psychological, and spiritual growth, all of my relationships change for the better. Some of them end, or morph into a different type of relationship, depending on if the other person is growing too, or growing in a similar way to me. If I continue to grow, and to treat others and myself with kindness, the transitions are never dramatic and don't create suffering.

Even so, sometimes it takes a while before you are sure of what wants to happen next. Perhaps you've been working on yourself, but your relationship hasn't shifted. You are in the "Should I stay or should I go" hallway, and you just want a door or window to open and show you the way. You could hang out in that hallway and suffer, or you could try a little something I call the Just Be Nice Campaign.

The Just Be Nice Campaign

When someone comes to me unsure if they should end a relationship or stick it out, I always suggest that they try *just being nice*. If that seems simple, it is. But sometimes simple is not easy. A big part of waking up is realizing how very simple life can actually be when we aren't stuck in the stories in our minds. Deepening simplicity in your life is a sure sign that you are on the right track.

So, how do we Just Be Nice? Well, there are a few simple instructions for the Just Be Nice Campaign:

1 Choose a period of time. I suggest ninety days. If that feels like too much for you, go with a shorter period that works for you, and really commit.

2 For that period of time, work on yourself and be the very best partner you can, regardless of how the other person is acting.

3 Just Be Nice to your partner. When they leave their balled-up socks all over the apartment, just be nice. When they guilt trip you about how many hours you are working, just be nice. When they do or say anything that bothers you, just be nice. This doesn't mean being treated like a doormat. You can state your needs and your boundaries (in a nice way). For any of the small things, and they are almost always small things, you don't always need to say a word. Just keep your side of the street clean.

4 Talk to friends, teachers, or therapists when you need to vent.

5 Plan fun things to do with your partner. Then do them and have fun, nicely.

6 Forgive yourself when you don't do this perfectly. Just keep doing your best every day, one day at a time.

7 At the end of the three months (or whatever amount of time you planned), you may have your answer regarding if you should stay or go. If you don't, restart the Just Be Nice Campaign.

I've done this myself a few times. I was just nice. When I got annoyed, scared, frustrated, felt not heard, got triggered—I was just nice. Sometimes that meant leaving the room for a moment, but no matter what, I was just nice. I focused on being the best partner I could be and took any focus off of what I thought the other person was doing wrong. I still spoke to someone and/or wrote about my feelings, but I didn't take problems or negativity to my partner. I got more clarity on what was actually a problem versus me simply being reactive.

Many of your complaints and criticisms about your partner don't actually need to be expressed. These are tiny issues that can actually be solved through just being nice. You can use **FOCUS ON SELF** to explore the uncomfortable feelings and thoughts. This gives you a chance to deconstruct the selves that arise in response to irritation or anger. There can be a lot of angry little selves that want you to believe them to be solid. They aren't. As you watch them crumble, most of the issues you have with your partner will crumble right along with them. When you don't point negative emotional energy at your partner, you get to actually look at it. You might find that you don't want to carry around all the negativity anymore.

Impermanent Conflict

I don't know anyone who *loves* conflict, but that doesn't mean it isn't necessary sometimes. Conflict is a natural occurrence in relationships and shouldn't be avoided just because it's uncomfortable. I find that it comes up when some part of the relationship is ready to expand and evolve. It's our job as mindful people to see past the surface of the conflict, into the underlying reasons behind it.

One of the reasons conflict is scary is because it reminds us that the relationship is not a solid, unmoving entity. It could change. It could end (spoiler alert: it *will* end one way or another). For some, even a little conflict triggers an end-of-the-world response. That's how I used to be. I couldn't tolerate even mild conflict in my relationships. When it inevitably came up, I would either crumple into a shut down mess, or try my best to destroy my opponent as if we were in a fight to the death, *Game of Thrones* style. I'm still working on how to be one hundred percent mindful in conflicts with my partners, but I've come a long way thanks to my meditation practice and skilled couple's therapists.

Impermanence is a fact of life, and it extends into your relationships. Your relationship is not permanent. Even in the best-case scenario, short of a freak accident that takes you both, one partner will eventually die, leaving the other one. Ideally, you and your partner will change over the years. If you're not changing, you're not growing. The ways you change won't always compliment the ways your partner does. There will be illnesses, deaths and births, career successes and failures, and hopefully many spiritual awakenings. All of this will create change in your relationship.

Here is a meditation designed to get you in touch with impermanence.

the practice

- Sit down and relax from your head to your toes.

- Practice BASIC BREATH AWARENESS, but pay special attention to the way the sensation of breathing moves and changes.

- Keep your focus on the changing quality of breath. Stay with this for a few minutes.

- Now shift your attention to include any kinds of sensations in the body that are moving and changing. This could include your heartbeat, a headache, or digestion. Notice how these sensations are not solid. They move and change. They flow.

- Try the same practice with your mind. Observe how the thoughts come and go. Thoughts are constantly moving and changing. Observe the impermanence.

This is a practice that is wonderful to do in nature with your eyes open. You can sit down and easily witness impermanence. The movement of leaves in the trees. The rustle of some furry creature in the bushes. The sounds of birds calling to one another. The workings of nature are a clear example of impermanence, and you only need look and listen to understand.

Once you are comfortable with impermanence, you no longer feel it necessary to cling so tightly to anything. You know on a deep level that everything is constantly changing. That includes ourselves, our partners, and our relationships. This helps make conflict feel less threatening. When you understand that everything is changing, you know that the conflict won't last forever. That makes a disagreement or awkward phase with your partner much less of a big deal. The phrase, *This too shall pass,* takes on true meaning, not just something people say when someone is going through a tough time.

No Problems, Only Solutions

As much as conflict can be a bummer, it can also be a sign that you are on the right track. Like I mentioned, conflict is often a sign that some expansion wants to occur. I've seen this in relationships, and also with individuals. For me, when I come up against a sense of conflict within myself, it means it's time to wake up and pay attention. If I stay present and mindful, it's easy to allow myself to grow through the conflict into the next version of me. Sometimes that can take minutes and sometimes it takes years, but eventually conflict gives way to something else. Again and again, you will see that there are no problems, only solutions, as John Lennon said.[3]

It's important to appreciate the tough times, but you don't want to become so accustomed to conflict that you can't grow without it. As a person who respects and appreciates conflict, I've needed to come to terms with my own attachment to it. There was a time that I created and gravitated toward conflict just to avoid myself. I drummed up a lot of melodramas in my heyday! Eventually, I had no interest in intentionally creating conflict, but the personal narrative I clung to was centered around how I was growing spiritually as a result of conflict.

Most of my conversations were about the challenges I had worked through, was currently working through, or would be soon working through. I deeply identified with my relationship to conflict and while it was helpful, it started to drain me. I still felt drawn to conflict because I believed that was what would make me grow the most, and the *fastest.*

A friend mentioned that I used the word *trauma* a lot and asked what it might be like if I dropped that word when talking about myself. It immediately struck a chord with me and I thanked him for pointing that out, and went about untangling from the self who was in love with personal growth through conflict. My recovery from trauma is one of my proudest accomplishments, but at some point you've got to set down your gloves and step out of the ring. Letting go of my attachment to conflict and my trial-by-fire personal growth attitude freed me up to have more joy and ease in my life.

Whether you are conflict-avoidant or totally attached to conflict, it can be hard to realize the potential of your relationships. Conflict is inevitable, but it's not constantly required. It's both something to open up to and something to let go of, depending on where you are. Be honest with yourself about what is needed for you.

When It Doesn't Work Out

Not all partners are going to be your forever person. Break-ups happen and so do broken hearts. The first time I had a broken heart was shocking and unbearable. I was seventeen and had been dating this guy I thought was really cool. He read obscure literature, listened to obscure music, and shot heroin. I would ride the train into the city to see him in the various one-bedroom apartments he shared with whoever would have him. I was really attached to this guy. He was kind enough, but being a drug addict made him perfect for my relationship pattern of choice. News flash: He didn't stop doing heroin out of his undying love for me and prove once and for all that I was loveable.

I was underage, so he would buy me beer. We would sit on the floor, smoke cigarettes, and seek mutual oblivion. We had been attempting a relationship for about a year when I, as he put it, "dropped the L-bomb." He informed me that while he enjoyed my company, love was the last thing on his mind. Looking back, it was the last thing on my mind too. I had no clue how to love myself, let alone anybody else. But at that time all I knew was that I was being rejected and it hurt like hell. All the parts of me that believed I was unlovable and inadequate came to life. I cried all night at his place, cried all the way home on the train, and walked into the apartment I shared with my dad, puffy, red, and still crying. My dad thought someone had died, and I felt sure it was going to be me.

For days I could barely move. The tears came in a torrential downpour. I couldn't believe how much it physically hurt. My chest felt hollow and filled with cement at the same time. The ache was so intense that I thought maybe a broken heart could actually kill me. My brain wouldn't shut up. It reminded me of how devastated I was, how "heartbroken" I was. Whenever I would start to feel better, there would be a surge of mental talk retriggering the intense physical sensations. I took everything my mind said personally; I believed all of it.

I needed to make it stop. I started calling friends, asking what to do. Everyone told me that I had a broken heart, and that the only thing to do was to wait it out. What no one told me was that suffering through a broken heart is totally optional. In addition, having a broken heart can supercharge your spiritual and emotional evolution.

After that first one, my breakups became more and more dramatic. Each time a relationship ended, no matter how dysfunctional, I would lose it. I would stop eating, stop sleeping, roll up in a ball on the floor for hours, make really creepy shrines in honor of my lost love, go on two-month-long pill popping, black out binges, create musical soundtracks to keep me as miserable as possible, drink until I could no longer actually get drunk, have really embarrassing rebound relationships, and tell the story of my broken heart over and over and over again to anyone who would listen. These symptoms could go on for months. I started very seriously considering suicide. I was suffering more than I could bear. At the same time, I was addicted to my suffering.

I Will Survive

Somewhere along the line, I started to dip my toes back into the meditation pool for the first time since I was a kid. Someone gave me the Pema Chödrön book, *When Things Fall Apart*. I began sitting for five minutes at a time, here and there. I noticed that there was a voice inside my head that wasn't very nice. I didn't yet understand that my body was full of sensations, many of them emotional. I felt the emotional pain in my chest and throat, but it was completely tangled up with my thoughts. After a while, those five-minute sits every once in a while became thirty to sixty minutes every day, and that's when my relationship with my mind and body changed dramatically.

About four years later, I had a chance to try out my new skills on a broken heart. What a difference a daily practice makes. Was I sad that my relationship hadn't worked out? Yes. Was there a lot of chatter in my mind about it? Yes. Did I experience unpleasant emotional sensations in my body? Yes. Did I suffer? No. Well, maybe a tiny bit, but we are talking about five minutes here and there. It was a huge difference. There was no pill popping or shrine building this time.

The night the breakup occurred I cried for a bit and meditated on the emotions in my chest and belly. Then I tried to get some sleep, but my mind was racing. It kept telling me all the things I could have done differently; all the things I should have said or not said. Over and over it replayed the final interactions with my now-absent lover. I would fall asleep and the mental talk would literally wake me up.

I did what I had been trained to do: mindfully attend to the mental talk with as much concentration, clarity, and equanimity as possible. I was amazed at how my brain created and re-created the problem. I was not asking my brain to do this (in fact, at moments when I lost my equanimity, I really wanted it to stop), but it kept going like a powerful computer, crunching the facts.

I also worked with the flow of the mental talk. It rose and fell in waves. It was very much like being rocked by the ocean. It started to become soothing instead of uncomfortable. It was waking me up, but it was also putting me back to sleep.

By five in the morning, when the talk woke me up for the fourth time, I laughed. It was hilarious and almost endearing or cute. Later, I talked with some close friends about the situation, but my mind was relatively quiet. I had let it do its computing, without judging it or resisting it. I knew that eventually I would get some sleep, and that the chatter would stop when it was ready to. By allowing it, but not taking it personally or wallowing in it, I had a complete experience of it. It passed through me and was gone.

As for the physical sensations, I enjoyed working with them. Emotions in my body tell me that I'm alive. I am learning to let go of attachments to "pleasant" or "unpleasant," and instead to explore sensation as sensation. Waves, vibration, heat, cold, contraction, expansion. When you mindfully contact the experience of a "hollow ache" or "physical exhaustion," without the mental label of "broken heart," it's just sensation.

Open Heart

I've had more than a few people ask me how meditation can help with the pains of a relationship ending. In my own experience, I've seen that it can help a lot. The main trick is learning to separate the emotional sensations in the body from the thoughts in the mind. You can do this by using **FOCUS ON SELF**. Once you can do that, you are able to deconstruct the sensations and the thoughts into smaller more manageable pieces. That's easier said than done in the midst of a broken heart, but with practice, you will find that it becomes automatic.

I got a lot out of that last broken heart. The emotional pain gave me direct access to some aspects of my consciousness that had been long buried. By fully allowing all my feeling and thoughts about the breakup to occur, I was able to heal much older wounds. I saw myself change very quickly during that time. I became more open, more available to others, less defensive, more alive. Really leaning into your meditation practice during tough times brings great rewards.

For a lot of us, a broken heart is very romantic. We see it in movies, hear it in songs, and revel in the drama of it. It can be so addictive. We have an idea of what it is like when our heart is broken and we hold tight to that idea. Our neural pathways are programmed. *This is what the end of a relationship should feel like. This is how I should behave.* We don't realize that there are many ways of experiencing a breakup, not all of which include big blow-outs and months of suffering.

For me, it was a matter of life and death to find a new way of being brokenhearted. Even if it's not that dire for you, why not try a new experience?

My relationship with the idea of a broken heart has changed. I have felt the emotions move through my body and vanish. If I get stuck in mental talk or put a value on the sensations in my body, then— bam!—I have a broken heart. If I simply and openly observe what is happening, it's just what's happening, one moment to the next.

One big insight that I gained from my last broken heart is this: *A broken heart is an open heart.* This sounds a little cheesy, I know, but it was true for me. When I fully experienced the many facets of my heartbreak, I found expansive open space. Instead of becoming jaded and afraid to love again, I realized that within all that space was room for more love than I ever imagined.

I'm not excited about the prospect of going through another big breakup. I hope I don't have to, but I know for sure that my heart will be broken again. This is part of being human. People you love will die. Natural disasters will occur. Wars will rage. You have a choice about how much you want to suffer and about how much you want to perpetuate suffering. Let your heart break open and meet life openly and with love.

Relationship as a Monastery

Shinzen Young talks about how if you choose to be in a romantic relationship, rather than celibate, it can serve as your own personal monastery.[4] You can do this by treating your relationship as sacred, and allowing it to be a container for your evolution. This is a way that you can, as a regular, nonmonastic person, develop a monastery. All you need to do is make your relationship a part of your spiritual practice. In the same way that you can bring mindfulness into washing the dishes or driving to work, you can bring mindfulness into your relationship. Aim to become more present and clear with each interaction. Find ways to incorporate more mindful communication into every day. Practice meditation together. And bring mindfulness into your sex life.

As we have explored thus far, there are so many ways to be mindful about sex and sexuality. If you want to create a monastery within your romantic relationship, sex is a great place to start. Begin to think of your sex life as a place to expand your limits and discover new ways of experiencing your spiritual life. Don't forget that mindful sex can be any kind of sex. It can be fucking, not just making love. You don't need to create a binary between spiritual sex and non-spiritual sex. It's all spiritual! The way you can tap into the inherent spirituality is by greeting all aspects of sex with mindfulness. It can be as simple as allowing yourself to breathe and relax into pleasure. Over time, with practice, mindful sex will become the only kind of sex you have.

Turning your relationship and sex life into a contemplative space won't always be easy. Being mindful and awake doesn't mean never making a mistake. Choosing to live and love with true mindfulness is a brave and vulnerable thing to do. You are opening your heart and mind to the world (and your lovers) in a beautiful way when you make a decision to wake up. Not just anyone will be able to partner with you once you begin this journey to awakening. You will be so bright, so free. You will be capable of loving and being loved with a gentle bravery and authenticity, and only those who are doing the same will be able to meet you in a partnership. This goes even for a casual affair. Your lovers will be living from a paradigm that matches yours, and true connection, however fleeting, will be the new normal.

When a relationship is like a monastery, you and your partner are each other's greatest teachers. I believe that people come together to experience a healing. This can be the case with any type of relationship, but it is especially true in romantic relationships. You can easily figure out what it is that wants to be healed in you by paying attention to your buttons—the buttons your partner is always pushing that can provoke a reaction. Those tender spots give us access to deep and unseen emotional wounds. If you are willing to be mindful and take your awareness past the surface sting of hurt feelings, your buttons will lead you straight to insight and healing.

You always have a choice: Do you want to have a pointless argument or use a moment of conflict to grow? You and your partner can help each other wake up by continuing to make the choice to grow. Each time you do this, you'll expand the possibilities for love and connection. Your monastery can give you a chance to do that every day.

the big O

Some say that every orgasm is an opportunity for *la petite mort*, or "the little death." We are experiencing little deaths all the time: the change of seasons, the end of a meal, falling asleep and then waking up from sleep, the loss of a relationship and/or the loss of singlehood—even the subtle ending of a sensation or thought, or the exhale of breath. We are constantly given opportunities to embrace impermanence and death, but orgasm may be one of my favorites. Orgasm doesn't just feel good. It teaches us about impermanence, grasping, attachment, and embodiment. *La petite mort* is also a moment of transcendence from normal human experience. The mind is overpowered by waves of sensation. Boundaries are blown out of the water. You die into the present moment, burning up in the ecstasy of all-encompassing pleasure.

And it feels good. Bringing mindfulness into your relationship and experience with The Big O only makes it better. However, orgasms can bring up challenges too. Shame, anxiety, insecurity, attachment, and grasping can all arise when relating to sexual pleasure. Luckily, you have a mindfulness practice that can guide you through these challenges.

Orgasmic Shame

When I discovered my clitoris around age twelve, I started masturbating with the goal of orgasm. The main thing I remember about those early orgasms is that I felt a lot of shame. While I hadn't been given any negative messages about masturbation from my parents, I did have some early sexual trauma that could have created that sense of shame. I would promise myself I'd never do it again, and then do it again (of course) and feel guilty. Eventually, I didn't consciously feel that it was wrong anymore, but those feelings of shame manifested as anxiety.

I hear from a lot of people that they had the same experience of shame around adolescent orgasms. For some, it was because of body shaming, religious beliefs, or sexual abuse. For others, it was just a feeling that it was wrong without any clear reason why. This sense of shame can carry over in all kinds of ways into your sex life as an adult. Getting mindful about the level of shame that you have around orgasm is an important step in waking up sexually. As you address your feelings of shame about orgasm, shame in other parts of your life may surface. This shame is being *revealed to be healed*. Your meditation practice can help you to gently reveal and radically heal the parts of you that feel ashamed.

It can be tempting to isolate yourself when you are experiencing shame. You may want to hide out and avoid sexual or even platonic interactions with your partner or friends. This is the last thing I would recommend. While time for yourself is important, cutting yourself off from the love and care of your support system will only make things worse. It takes a lot of vulnerability to open yourself to others when the shame cycle is turned on, but talking to someone you love and trust can be a step toward feeling better.

Healing shame requires a truckload of self-love. Generally, the shame seed is planted early in life, and the shame you experience stems back to that original core wounding. You can use **FOCUS ON SELF** to get clarity on where the shame currently resides in your mind and body. When you locate the thoughts and emotions that correlate with your feelings of shame, greet them with acceptance, friendliness, and curiosity. The more acceptance and love you offer yourself in these areas, the better. Don't shame your shame away. Love yourself so much that the shame transforms. The part of us that feels shame needs to be loved and accepted just as it is. We all too often want to get rid of the parts of ourselves that experience emotions like shame, envy, or judgment. If instead we allow these aspects of self to be seen and cared for, we open up the possibility of true healing.

You can try this version of the **POSITIVITY BOOST** when dealing with shame.

—

the practice

- When you are aware of feelings of shame arising, take a comfortable seat. You can also lie down if that feels more supportive.

- Locate where you feel the shame in your body.

- Now rub your hands together, creating warmth between them. Then, place your hands on the parts of your body where you feel the sensations of shame.

- Use gentle pressure to soothe yourself.

- Now try saying these words to yourself: I see you and I love and accept you unconditionally.

- Continue to say these words as you offer yourself compassionate touch.

- If you can't locate the emotional sensations of shame, just place your hands on your belly and your heart and say the loving words.

- Practice this for as long as you like.

You can also try this practice just before having sex. You will be amazed how even five minutes of compassionate self-touch and positive affirmation can help you to let go of orgasmic shame and dive into orgasmic bliss.

You are not your shame. When we identify with things like shame, envy, and greed, we suffer. You are so much more than your shame, and your emotional experience includes a vast array of colors, some quite delightful. Don't limit yourself to the tiny box that shame can put you in. Expand beyond those finite thoughts and emotions and see yourself as you really are—limitless and free.

Orgasm Anxiety Be Gone

Anxiety is one of the top reasons people contact me for help. In my opinion, we have an anxiety epidemic going on: So many people are incredibly freaked out by money, health, sex, or the pressure to be perfect. The good news is that meditation can help immensely. Even Western doctors are starting to suggest meditation as a solution for anxiety. I can report that meditation has been a real anxiety-killer for me. One place that anxiety showed up for me was during sex, specifically in relation to orgasms. I was always worried that I wasn't coming fast enough. Through teaching about mindful sex, I have found out that many people deal with similar anxieties. The first guy I had sex with (the one with the ponytail) went down on me. I didn't understand what he was doing, and I didn't have an orgasm. I had heard of blowjobs, but not *that*. The next time I had

good sex tip

If the orgasm shame you carry with you is a result of some kind of abuse, it's imperative that you get very competent support in this area. A meditation practice is a good foundation for working with this material, but it's not always enough. A good therapist, a loving community, and safe, mindful partners are also key. Don't be afraid to seek the help and support that you need.

sex, my partner tried to bring me to orgasm with his hand. It felt good, but I froze up as soon as I realized that he had an end goal in sight. I got caught in my mind and couldn't seem to return to the pleasurable sensations. I felt like I was taking too long and he was getting bored with me. I felt like I was "doing it wrong." This was the beginning of my experience with orgasm anxiety.

I went on to fake every orgasm I ever had with my first boyfriend. I wasn't quite as convincing as Meg Ryan's famous scene in *When Harry Met Sally*, but looking back I don't think he cared either way. I don't think he actually liked vaginas. When that relationship ended, I was adamant that I would never again fake an orgasm. I'm happy to report that since then I never have. If you are faking it, stop. It doesn't do you or your partner any favors. You deserve so much more than a climax charade.

While I no longer pretended to get off, what did remain for some time was orgasm anxiety. I felt a huge amount of pressure to come and come fast. My mind would race, and the more it raced the less connected I would be with the pleasure in my body or my partner. I would worry that my partner didn't really want to be doing what they were doing. I imagined them thinking, *Oh god. When is this going to end?* Though I doubt these fantasies were reality, I felt rushed and judged—not a great combination for getting off or connecting with your partner. Orgasms had become, in effect, a problem.

At some point in my late teens I came up with a technique for getting out of my head and into my body. I would visualize that my brain was in my vagina and rather than thoughts, it manifested sensations. I would focus on those sensations, which would intensify the pleasure and give me some freedom from my mind. I wasn't a pro at this technique, but when I was able to employ it, my sex life was much improved. At the time I didn't realize that I was really on to something. I had discovered the beginnings of mindful sex for myself.

Here is a version of that technique that people who are having trouble with orgasm anxiety can try during sex.

—

the practice

- When moving toward orgasm, start by practicing breathing while contracting and releasing your pelvic floor muscles.

- This will help you move your attention to the pelvic area. Keep your full attention on this area.

- Anytime you get pulled into thoughts, bring your attention right back to your genitals.

- Continue to breathe and contract and release the pelvic floor.

- Remember to release, not just contract.

- Use your physical awareness to explore the sensations in your pelvic area.

- Get especially interested in pleasure. Soak into the pleasurable sensations, returning whenever you get pulled into thought.

With this simple technique, you can take the emphasis off of your thoughts and put it on feeling good.

Don't Think about Baseball

For people with penises whose orgasm anxiety is about coming too soon, FOCUS ON SELF can be a very helpful technique. As with any anxiety, orgasm anxiety can build upon itself until you become overwhelmed. If instead you can learn to deconstruct the thoughts and emotions related to your cjaculation anxiety, you will find that it loses its power to take you over.

Men are sometimes told to think about other things to keep from coming too early. To me this smacks of resistance—and resistance rarely works. Even worse, it's hard to practice mindful sex if you're thinking about something else the whole time, like baseball or your mother-in-law.

Instead, try slowing down and extending your foreplay sessions. Take time to fool around while you and your partner still have your clothing on. While you are having sex, tell your partner when you are getting close to climax and change positions or take a short break to just breathe and feel your body. This is sometimes called the "Start-Stop" method and, if done mindfully, can help to extend intercourse. Try the Start-Stop method on your own first and use BASIC BODY AWARENESS to get clear on the sensations that occur shortly before an orgasm. When you are comfortable with this method, try it with your partner. Be patient with yourself and ask your partner to help you stick with it.

Also, remember that intercourse isn't the only way to get it on. There are a lot of fun and pleasurable sex activities that don't require an erect penis. Exploring other aspects of sex will prove to be fun *and* hot for you and your partner.

I have come across many people who have some version of the orgasm anxiety that I experienced. I've known people who gave up altogether on having orgasms with their partners because of it and people who are so anxious about coming too soon that they avoid sex altogether. However, I've seen that for most people, bringing mindfulness into sex can help.

A New Story

An important step toward anxiety-free orgasms is to let go of the story that you've created: that you can't climax, or that you'll climax too soon, or that you can only climax within a very specific set of guidelines. This is just a story that you have been telling yourself—it is not necessarily true. You can stop listening to that story and write a new one.

Letting go of a belief you have carried for a long time is a process. Begin by noticing whenever that story pops into your head. Then, you can redirect and reframe your thoughts around orgasms. Try taking an anxious thought and flipping it to make a positive affirmation. Use this affirmation each day and while having sex if those anxious thoughts come up. This is how you'll be able to rewrite that tired old tale about not being able to orgasm.

You will also want to take apart the strands of experience that create the anxiety. Any ideas you have about yourself are composed of thoughts and emotions. That mental and emotional experience changes constantly and does not make up the whole of who you are. Deconstructing your orgasm anxiety will lower your suffering and increase your enjoyment and ease in getting frisky with your lover. This is not a small thing. The ability to decrease suffering here will extend to other parts of your life. Again and again, you can see how bringing mindfulness into your sex life improves your whole life.

Putting It into Practice

As you let go of anxiety and lean into enjoyment, being self-centered will go a long way. I don't mean thinking about yourself or being selfish in a negative way. I simply mean putting the focus on your own experience. I find that all too often folks are focused on their partner in an anxious way. *Are they enjoying this? Do they like the way I smell? Do they think I'm fat? Is this as good as it was with their ex?* If instead you focus on what is happening in your own body, practicing embodiment, you begin to get grounded in the present moment. Not surprisingly, as you drop into yourself you will begin to connect more deeply with your partner. A kind of sexual instinct will begin to arise.

This sexual instinct can be the new normal, leaving anxious lovemaking in the dust. As always, be patient and let go of trying to "get it right." When you first start to address your orgasm anxiety you might temporarily notice it more than ever. This can happen with any negative thought pattern or behavior that you become aware of. I've heard Pema Chödrön call this experience "heightened neurosis."[1] While this may seem problematic at first, it's actually a good sign. It means that you are waking up to the level of anxiety you have been tolerating. When you see the anxiety clearly, you can start to unwind from it and get free. Connect with your partner during this process. Let them in on what you are working through. They might be able to help.

Voicing your orgasm anxiety to your partner is very helpful. Try talking about it when you are not having sex—over breakfast or during an evening walk. Sharing your fears and insecurities about getting off will most likely be a big relief and a great chance for more intimacy with your partner. Be mindful of how you communicate on either end of this conversation. Especially in

good sex tip

For people on medications with sexual side effects, taking the emphasis off orgasm (and erection and vaginal lubrication) can be a real lifesaver. Rather than spending your time focused on what is not available, appreciate what is. There are lots of enjoyable aspects of sex, even without orgasm. You may even find that once you take the pressure off, it becomes easier to climax. Also, be sure to tell your doctor about sexual side effects; they are not considered insignificant. Your doctor may want you to try a different dose or medication.

the beginning, it can feel scary to talk about or hear about orgasm anxiety. Stay in touch with what is happening in your body and don't try to push a solution. Just beginning this conversation is a big and important step.

You and your partner can work as a team to reduce orgasm anxiety and increase enjoyment and connection. Some gentle and encouraging words during sex can go a long way to ease anxiety. The reframing of negative self-talk I mentioned earlier can be really powerful if said out loud by your partner. When your partner is whispering affirmations to you, it becomes easier to relax into the moment.

Orgasm Attachment

When I was a teenager, I read a news story about the musician Sting. He practiced Tantric sex and could go for seven hours. This made him (and his wife!) seem like sexual superheroes to me, but it wasn't until recent years that I actually started to investigate what is called Tantric sex in America. I discovered that Tantric sex practices can help with learning to relax during sex, and they can also help to soften our attachment to orgasm.

In Tantric sex, all the emphasis is on the energetic connection rather than the orgasm. In fact, you are encouraged not to focus on orgasm at all. This is a big change for most people, and requires a total rewiring of how we think about sex.

Because of my early experience with faking it and my vow to get mine, I was very attached to my orgasms. We humans move toward what feels good; it's how we are built. What I didn't realize is that all that expectation of what was to come was limiting my ability to be present for what was happening in the moment.

I was also attached to my partner's orgasms, and didn't feel satisfied if they hadn't come. A lot of that had to do with my issues of self-worth. If I didn't make them come, I wasn't good. Wasn't lovable. When I was with a partner who didn't overvalue orgasm, I felt very uncomfortable. It was actually more unsettling if I came and my partner didn't than the other way around. How could I make them like me if I didn't get them off?

Mindfulness leaves no stone unturned, and my attachment to orgasm had no chance of not being addressed. As I focused my practice more on my sex life and sexuality, I recognized a lot of grasping and unconscious material around orgasm.

Getting Off without Getting Off

Not getting off can be very challenging at first. Our attachments to orgasm can run deep, touching old emotional wounds and negative thought patterns. It can take some time and practice to find more equanimity with orgasm, but you'll be glad you did.

It can be helpful to play around with yourself before experimenting with a partner. Schedule a chunk of time when you have privacy and don't have to rush off anywhere afterward. Set the intention to create pleasure without climaxing.

___

the practice

- Set a timer for the desired time. Lie down and relax from your head to your toes.

- When you are ready, begin to touch your genitals. Don't jump into doing what you always do.

- If you are highly orgasmic be very mindful of not orgasming out of habit. Any gender can use the Start-Stop method.

- Move slowly and keep your body relaxed. Focus your attention on all of the various sensations arising in your body.

- Use the BASIC BODY AWARENESS and PLEASURE BOOST techniques.

- Notice when the desire to climax comes up.

- Use the FOCUS ON SELF technique to explore your thoughts and emotions.

- As your body becomes more aroused you may become incredibly desperate to give up on the exercise. At this point, you may want to stop touching your genitals and focus on that feeling of grasping.

- You may even notice some sadness or grief come up. Take a few moments to gently and mindfully attend to that before continuing to masturbate.

- Make sure to save some time at the end to again focus on the thoughts and emotions that arise when you don't climax.

- After you are done, do some stream of consciousness writing about what came up for you and how you feel masturbating without orgasm.

Get curious about what you find doing this exercise. Even a subtle emotion or whisper of a thought could be significant. It's easy to rush over insights and lose the possibility for evolution when we are striving to better ourselves sexually or otherwise. Take your time and thoroughly explore this new territory of sexual pleasure without the happy ending.

It's the Journey, Not the Destination

Having lovers that are as dedicated to waking up as I am made this shift to orgasmic equanimity much easier for me. At that time my partner enjoyed getting off, but didn't *need* to and often wouldn't. While this was challenging given my self-worth issues, it also made my work easier because more light was being shone on that once unconscious material. It was inspiring and healing to be with someone who could take or leave orgasms. Together we explored coming and not coming. Willing and loving partners will make sex more fun and enlightening every time.

Having sex without the focus being on orgasm can be a downright magical experience. When we are no longer stuck on where we are going, we can be where we are. Sex comes to life in a beautiful way. It has the opportunity to become more playful, more edgy, or more sensual. A kind of mystery starts to unfold when we don't have a destination in mind. I found that being surprised by what my body would do next was a heck of a lot more fun than sticking with the same old routines. My body continues to surprise me all of the time.

Spend hours fooling around like teenagers or have super slow sex. It can be fun to tease each other, or just let go of orgasm altogether and let your bodies merge in whatever way they want. Time can fly by pretty quickly doing this and you can find yourself in Sting territory before you know it!

Be Here Now

Taking orgasm out of the picture can reveal parts of the picture that you don't like. When sex is all about getting off we can gloss over areas that are unsatisfactory. As orgasm moves out of the spotlight, you may start to see that your sex life needs some work. Open, honest, and *loving* communication is imperative at this point. Everyone wants to be a good lover and feelings can be easily hurt. Get a coach or therapist to help with these conversations if it's too overwhelming to have them on your own. Though it may be uncomfortable at first, this is the beginning of a beautiful new stage of your relationship.

Orgasms are great, but there is more to sex than climax. As you learn to soak into pleasure and find deeper connection with your partner through the flow of sensation, any particular end result seems less important. You may find there are other kinds of sexual satisfaction when you are less attached to a specific outcome. It's completely possible that you could find yourself sprawled out, sweaty, vibrating with afterglow, exhausted, and totally satisfied—without ever having a traditional orgasm.

This exploration of taking the emphasis off of orgasm affects other aspects of life as well. How often are you doing something and focused only on the end result? How much more could you be getting out of even mundane everyday activities if you were not living in the future?

Your meditation practice will point you back to Now and help you cultivate an active relationship with the present moment. The exploration of orgasm can be the vehicle that leads you to being more present.

Orgasm and Concentration

When I'm working with a student and they say, "I really liked that technique. It was fun and it felt good," I always suggest that they continue to practice in that way. When you have a good time with your meditation practice, you are much more likely to keep up your practice. The benefit of choosing to work with a technique that you enjoy is that it becomes easy to drop into a deep and highly pleasurable kind of concentration.

Have you ever been totally lost in a sunset, or a kiss? With meditation, you can train yourself to be that concentrated on something as simple as your breath. Everything else will fall away as your attention gathers around just this inhale and just this exhale, for long stretches of time. It's an incredibly centered and simple feeling, and at the same time rich with life and pleasure. It's a ravishing peace of the mind and body. There are deeper and deeper levels of this kind of concentration. But you don't need to drop into that kind of concentration to enjoy the bliss of being focused. An orgasm delivers you right into a deeply concentrated state.

All focus goes to the waves, spikes, and tingles of pleasure coursing through your body. You get a short version of the benefits of meditation for free with each orgasm. People spend years trying to attain this level of concentration, not realizing that a crash course is available in their next climax, if they pay attention.

Consider this. Do you find yourself thinking *during* an orgasm? Perhaps this is one of the reasons we love our orgasms. They give us a break from being so preoccupied with the stories in our minds. People who have a meditation practice and have strong concentration skills can get even more out of this moment of bliss.

You can get a taste for this type of concentration with your very next orgasm. Try it on your own first, and then try it with a partner.

---

the practice

- Use **BASIC BODY AWARENESS** to practice Mindful Masturbation.

- As you are nearing orgasm, find stillness in as much of the body as possible.

- Focus all your attention on the genital area. Use the tools of **PLEASURE BOOST**.

- As the pleasure increases it will be easier and easier to sustain your concentration.

- Stay present as you tip over into full climax, noticing how everything else falls away.

- Do your best to continue to concentrate in this way even after your orgasm has ended.

- Use the momentum of the orgasm to stay with the subtle waves of pleasure and hum of sensation for as long as you can.

Using orgasm to sensitize yourself to deep concentration can help you to recognize it and nurture it in your meditation practice. The ability to concentrate for even short bursts will extend into longer periods. I like telling my students that having highly developed concentration skills is like having a superpower. You can do things better and feel better while you do them. Even a monotonous task can become interesting and pleasurable if you are deeply concentrated on it.

The more concentrated you are, the more present you can be. The more present you are, the more awake you are. This concentrated wakefulness is an important stage on the spiritual path, but don't get down on yourself if your concentration skills are not the best. My teacher, Adyashanti, tells a story of how he was never a good meditator because he couldn't concentrate. That didn't keep him from waking up, going on to teach around the globe, and getting married to another teacher of mine, his wife, Mukti.

Practice kindness with yourself as you strengthen your concentration skills. You are training your brain and that takes time. Relax your body as you concentrate, and celebrate the growth whenever you notice that your focus has improved. It's important not to get too attached to your techniques for concentration. Eventually, all technique will want to fall away as you simply sit with the majestic flow of experience.

eight
press play

Please note: This chapter discusses sexual abuse.

Let's look at how much money America alone spends on porn each year. According to figures calculated by California's state legislature, the U.S. porn industry rakes in approximately $11 billion annually. That's a lot of porn, and it doesn't count the millions of people watching "free" porn on sites like XTube or PornHub. So we can agree that many people watch porn, including "spiritual" people. I think it's high time we start bringing our spiritual practice to our use of porn. I think this type of content has the ability to aid in our sexual awakening and deepen our connection with our partners. So let's talk about porn.

While I don't identify as a Buddhist, I do attend Buddhist meditation retreats at least once a year. At these meditation retreats everyone is asked to follow the Buddhist precepts, a list of the values and ethics of Buddhism. The precepts are already a part of my personal philosophy, so it's never a big deal for me to agree to them while on retreat. As a sex-positive and nontraditional person the third precept is an important one for me. This precept asks that we avoid sexual misconduct. That can mean different things for different people. For me it translates as *Do No Harm*. No harm to others and no harm to myself. You can follow the third precept and be non-monogamous. You can follow the third precept and like to tie your partner up and strike their bare bottom with a flogger. You can follow the third precept and watch porn or even make it. What's important is how you do these things. Is there full consent and protection for all involved? Are you clear on your intentions and motives? Are you mindful and kind? Bringing the third precept or a similar philosophy into your sexual life can be a gift to yourself and your partners.

This philosophy of *Do No Harm* continues to evolve and deepen for me. As I mature and awaken on new levels so does my understanding of what constitutes sexual misconduct. One area in which I experienced a big shift was with pornography. I don't watch porn that often, but now and then I enjoy it and I think it's a great tool for exploring sexuality. However, in the past I would watch anything that turned me on. I didn't think much about the performers involved, or how they were being treated in the industry. I wasn't conscious of the suffering that was being perpetuated by some of the content I was viewing. It was much like when I ate meat without any thought for the animals that suffered or for the terrible environmental impact caused by the meat industry. Once I fully embraced the truth about eating animals, my diet changed drastically. When my body needs animal protein I spend the money to buy meat that comes from ethical sources. The same kind of thing happened with my feelings about porn. And once you have a moment of clarity about something like this, it changes you. For me, that moment of clarity came from watching Rashida Jones' documentary *Hot Girls Wanted*.[1] While this film has been criticized by the porn industry, including people in it who felt exploited and mistreated by the production company, it had a big effect on me. After seeing it, I could no longer watch porn that wasn't ethical.

I am now much more mindful about my relationship with porn. I encourage anyone who fancies naughty videos to take the time to do the same. Do you watch ethical porn? Do you feel shame about enjoying porn? Can you talk to your partner about porn, or even enjoy it with them? These are all questions to ask yourself.

I like porn. I believe that someone who is spiritual can also enjoy porn. Of course all porn is not created equal. It's important to know where your porn comes from and how it is made. Life is not black and white; it's all gray area. It's our job as people who hope to evolve to see these shades of gray. Just because you meditate doesn't mean you can't enjoy a rough BDSM (Bondage and Discipline/ Domination and Submission/Sadism and Masochism) scene or a book of erotic photography. Because you meditate, you'll be able to enjoy porn more, and with less attachment. If porn is triggering for you, I still invite you to read this section. Stay in touch with your thoughts and emotional sensations as you read. No one says you have to watch this kind of content, but having an aversion to it can create unnecessary suffering for yourself.

When I was a kid I was a bit of a snoop and figured I'd find something good if I looked on the top shelf of an older family member's closet. I found dust, some loose change, and a healthy stack of dirty magazines. It was like finding a new planet or species. Women like I had never seen, with tiny waists and massive breasts, spread themselves over the thick pages. They had strangely groomed pubic hair that looked very different from my mom's. They had juicy red lips and long pointy finger nails, like some kind of mythical creatures. Some of them were touching their vaginas, spreading the lips open. They all looked back at me from the glossy paper with coy smiles and pleasure-filled eyes. I *had* to show my siblings what I had found! We spent a few weeks sneaking into the room and laying the magazines out on the floor. Silently we feasted our eyes on the skin, lace, round bottoms, and arched backs. (I was particularly fond of the jokes too. I had a mature sense of humor for a nine-year-old.) Eventually our secret got out and the magazines disappeared from my life as quickly as they had entered.

What I remember most about that experience is the joy and discovery I felt. These women were like nothing I had ever seen. They made my body feel something it had never felt. It was beyond exciting to see into this new world. I still think of porn that way. It's a peek into another human's sexual expression. A glimpse past the conventions of our puritan culture that is afraid of sex and nudity. A feeling of connection with the people who are sharing their bodies, pleasure, and personality. Pornography at its best can educate, inspire, and heal us.

I can already hear the angry thoughts some of you are having as you read this. Don't you fear, I most likely agree with everything you are thinking. Porn at its worst can exploit, misinform, and cause actual harm and suffering to humans. This is true, but it is not the only truth. Just like there is healthy food and unhealthy food there is healthy porn and unhealthy porn. Sadly, I would guess that a great percentage of the content that people are viewing is of the unhealthy variety. By unhealthy, I don't mean the content of the porn per se. Some of the most intense BDSM porn I've viewed has also been some of the most ethical. As long as you are watching consenting adults in ethical porn, I say enjoy whatever kind of content you want. The good news is that it doesn't take much work to find ethical porn.

Ethical Porn

What is ethical porn you ask? Ethical porn is content (including films, photography, webcams, etc.) in which the performers are fully consenting to the material. Ethical porn pays their performers well and protects their health and safety above all. Ethical porn can be performer-owned and operated, based on an individual's own sexual creativity. Ethical porn can be any kind of porn as long as all parties are treated with kindness, care, and the utmost respect. Ethical porn usually isn't free. Ethical porn is the only kind of porn we should be watching.

It is so easy to access sexual content online today. Pre-internet, the best you could get was a scrambled cable channel with the odd breast or penis visible. Even when the world wide web came along, it was dial-up and it took forever to load just a few minutes of video. Now porn is available at your fingertips anytime you want, fancy, fast and free. This is where we must consider, *Is this content ethical? Does is fall within my understanding of* Do No Harm? It's easy to brush aside your conscience with a justification, but you must be willing to look at the bigger picture. Even if you are paying for your porn, it's your job to make sure it comes from a reputable source. Living a mindful and awakened life means being mindful and awake even when it's more convenient not to be. To make sure your porn is ethical, the number one thing to do is *pay for it.* Another way to be mindful of your content is to look for before-and-after videos of the performers stating their consent, and often pleasure and joy. You can also find performers on social media and take note of what scenes they are tweeting about. If a performer is posting about a film or production company, it's highly likely that they had a good experience. If you want to offer some extra support you can often find performer wishlists or the option to tip.

Here's how Tristan Taormino, feminist, author, educator, and activist, explains ethical porn:

> Ethical porn shares many values with feminist pornography, and there is a great deal of overlap. Makers of ethical porn are committed to a fair and ethical production process,

which can include: fair wages to performers (performers set their rates and producers don't bargain) and fair hours; compliance with all laws regarding age verification and worker safely and protection; an environment that supports and values sex workers for the work they do; providing performers with all the tools they need, including their choice of safer sex materials, lube, sex toys as well as food and beverages; and encouraging authentic experiences of desire, pleasure, and orgasm. Respect is essential on an ethical porn set and consent is explicit and ongoing, so performers have the agency to make decisions about everything they do; their physical, sexual, and psychological well being is prioritized. If you care where your food or clothing comes from and the conditions under which it is made, then you should care where your porn comes from. Ethical and feminist porn are like organic, fair-trade products.

good sex tip

If you really want to be 100 percent sure that your porn is cruelty-free, make your own! Most phones are equipped with a great video camera these days. Entire feature films are filmed on iPhones now, so whether you're an amateur or not you can certainly make a decent "sex tape." It can either be a spontaneous shoot or something you plan out (or even enlist friends to get involved with). The making of your personal porn will be its own fun sex adventure—and you get to watch it! Keep in mind that even if you have friends setting the lighting and shooting the scene, your DIY porn probably won't look like the professional version. Enjoy the homemade quality and don't get caught up in getting it perfect. Remember: Anything you put online could be released to the world. Unless you don't mind other people getting off to your porn, keep it on a hard drive, not the Cloud.

The great thing about doing your research and choosing to only watch ethical porn is that afterward you can just sit back and enjoy. For me, knowing that my porn isn't causing suffering allows me to get way more pleasure from viewing it. You can let go of any guilt or judgment and go along for the ride. If you feel drawn to exploring porn as a part of your sexuality, let go of the idea that a "spiritual person" wouldn't do that. You get to decide what is right for you. In the back of the book I've listed resources for ethically-made porn. Enjoy!

Porn and Shame

I'm passionate about discussing sex so openly because, as Brené Brown says in her famous TED Talk, "Vulnerability is the antidote to shame."[2] I've come to learn that the more transparent and vulnerable I am, the less shame I experience. I think that sexual shame is one of the top Good Sex killers, and sadly so many of us are plagued by it. People's relationship with porn is an area where a ton of this shame can reside. Moving through it requires opening up and getting honest with ourselves and others. But shame can be disorienting and cause us to freeze up, cutting off honest self inquiry. So let's deconstruct the shame associated with viewing porn!

Writing is an incredibly powerful tool for dismantling and healing shame. Whenever I become aware of some unresolved shame, I put pen to paper and hash it out. Here are a few questions for you to explore in some stream of consciousness writing:

1. When do I first remember becoming aware of porn?

2. How did I feel about porn when I first became aware of it?

3. What messages did I get from parents and other adults about porn?

4. What do I think of people who watch porn?

5. What do I think of people who make or perform in porn?

6. What kind of porn turns me on? (Or what kind do I think might?)

7. How do I feel in my body after viewing porn?

8. What are some bad experiences, if any, I have had involving porn?

9. What are some good experiences, if any, I have had involving porn?

10. Do I think watching porn is bad or unspiritual? If so, why?

Once you've explored all or some of these questions in writing, take some time to practice **FOCUS ON SELF**. Notice what thoughts and emotions come up and offer them acceptance. If you are feeling overwhelmed, switch to **REST AND RELAX** for a bit until this emotion passes.

The next step is to talk honestly about your thoughts and feelings regarding porn. Choose someone you trust who will listen and not pass judgment. If you have a partner perhaps you will have this talk with them; or maybe a close friend or therapist would be best. The point here isn't to figure anything out, but instead to just begin a conversation. One of the best ways to eradicate shame is to talk openly.

You may find that a lot of your shame around porn was actually inherited from your parents, your religion, or your culture in general. If you were raised to think sex is wrong, dirty, or reserved only for married people, it's easy to see why you might feel bad about yourself for watching sexual content. In some cases, while sex isn't vilified, it simply isn't discussed. As you grow up and start to experiment, the influence of your culture will color your beliefs about sex, and thus about porn too.

In general, there is a negative attitude toward porn. One main complaint I hear is how porn affects teenagers' sexuality and their sexual interactions. I don't argue that this isn't an issue, but blaming all porn doesn't actually get to the heart of the matter. I believe that if these young people were educated about sex *and* porn in a positive and non-shameful way, the result would be very different.

Kids and Porn

Not that long ago an old friend of mine contacted me about her daughter. She was eleven years old and had been getting in trouble at school for talking about sex. Then my friend discovered a bunch of hardcore porn sites in her daughter's browser history. She was understandably concerned as her daughter was so young and the content was so intense.

My first suggestion was to sit down with her daughter and discuss the sexual values that she wanted to pass along. I advised that she lay out the whole enchilada: sexual pleasure, the pros and cons of having sex as a teen, STIs, and pregnancy. I also suggested that my friend talk with her daughter about porn. Maybe even explain to her that once she's older, she could explore the options of ethical porn: porn in which the performers are consenting, paid well, and treated with respect. I invited her to explain the difference between ethical porn and everything else. That it's important to choose wisely when deciding what to watch. I suggested that my friend ask her daughter if she had any questions about sex. I invited my friend to try her best to listen without judgment, and to respond as openly and positively as she could. I also added that the conversation was an important one to have and would shape her daughter's view of sex and sexuality.

I think it's incredibly important to have these talks with children and teens. If they understand that porn isn't "real," that it's a performance, they are much less likely to think that sex is supposed to look like that all the time. When sex and porn aren't treated like some secretive, shameful topic, I believe that kids will have a much healthier relationship with their own sexuality. Talking to kids (and adults) about ethical porn as an alternative to sites like Porn-Hub will give them the chance to make conscious choices when it comes to the content they view.

Body Image

Talking openly about porn will also help soothe unrealistic body expectations that can come up. You are not expected to look like a porn star, folks! For the most part, porn features people who have exaggerated good looks and exaggerated body parts. But even porn stars don't look like porn stars all the time. Makeup, good lighting, post-production work, and in some cases, plastic surgery, all play a part in the finished product. Don't judge yourself based on someone who is in front of the camera for a living.

I'm an actor and model and let me tell you, airbrushing and Photoshop can do wonders. When I show up on set in my sweatpants with sleepy eyes I look nothing like I do in the film or final photograph. I have cellulite and wrinkles just like most women my age, and the performers you see in porn are not perfect either. Not to mention we are all human, which means we are all going to get old (if we are lucky) and die. When I'm feeling envious of a twenty-something with smooth skin and no gray hair, I remind myself that they will one day be my age, and that makes me feel a little better!

If you find that watching mainstream porn is making you feel bad about yourself, try exploring indie or "real people" porn. Not everyone wants to see "perfect" breasts and huge penises, so there is a huge variety out there. Personally, the traditional porn star look doesn't really do it for me. I prefer watching real people have real sex. Tumblr is a great place to find homemade porn from adventurous people, which is often ethical and free!

At the end of the day, good sex always includes feeling good about yourself. Your body is totally desirable and beautiful just the way it is. The more unconditional love and acceptance you offer yourself, the better your sex life will be. If porn doesn't add to your attitude of self-love then don't watch it.

Your Relationship on Porn

Another area in which I hear complaints about porn is within the context of monogamous relationships. For the most part I hear from women who are uncomfortable with their male partners watching porn, though I've heard it from others too. Some go so far as to consider viewing porn as cheating. If this is something you are struggling with, it's important to get crystal clear on what is actually bothering you. Until you suss out exactly why your partner's porn consumption is a problem for you, there will be no resolution.

For some, it comes down to simple insecurity. If your partner is getting sexually aroused by anyone other than you, you must not be good enough. This is of course not even a little bit true. Your self-worth is not measured by your partner's attraction to someone else, or the fact that some porn turns them on. Self-worth comes from within, by way of self-love and acceptance, not through any outside person, place, or thing. Rather than judging your partner's sexuality or sexual preference, take a look at how you can practice more self-soothing and love. Also let your partner know how you feel! Don't put down their proclivity for porn; instead be vulnerable and share your insecurity. Everyone feels insecure sometimes, and if your partner is mindful and conscious they will be able to set you at ease.

Jealousy can also create issues with porn use in relationships. I delve into working with jealousy in Chapter Fourteen, but I'd like to touch lightly on it now. Jealousy, in my experience, is always hiding something deeper. Usually this is a fear of abandonment, which can stem from experiences early on in life or from past relationship trauma. It is your responsibility to address these deeper issues. A good partner can help if you allow them to see what's at the core of your jealousy, but you'll need to do the heavy lifting. **FOCUS ON SELF** is a great way to get under the surface of your jealousy and find out what's really going on. By taking apart the strands of experience that make up jealousy, you'll be able to access the tender places inside that need to heal. For me, working through jealousy was incredibly transformative, albeit painful at times.

Cultural shame can also influence your opinions about your partner, or yourself, watching porn. If you've been told that porn is "bad" and "dirty," then you may have adopted this stance unconsciously. Be sure that your past programming isn't negatively affecting your present-day relationship. Get clear on how your beliefs have been formed and decide if they are actually serving you and your partner.

If you've already addressed your own jealousy, insecurities, and any culturally-induced shame but still have a problem with your partner's porn use, it may be time to take a long, hard look at the relationship. Do you and your partner share the same values? Are your sexual selves compatible? Is this just one issue or the tip of the iceberg? Your issues with porn might just be the place where you are putting all the negative energy that actually resides in many other places. Before ending a relationship, I suggest trying couples therapy or counseling first. Also, don't rule out the possibility that porn could actually be used to build intimacy and connection.

Porn for Intimacy

Porn can, in fact, deepen intimacy and connection with your partner when it's being used in a mindful way. It's a vulnerable thing to talk about porn and watch it together, but vulnerability always creates more intimacy (and better sex!). When I was younger I had a lot of insecurity about being turned on by porn. When I did watch porn with a partner I had to push through a ton of discomfort and that resulted in a lack of presence and mindfulness on my part. I felt shame that porn turned me on but I wasn't willing to address that with myself or my partner. As I mentioned earlier, being open about shame and embracing vulnerability is the gateway to healing and intimacy. As I grew emotionally and spiritually I began sharing my inner world with my partners; now porn is a fun and sexy ingredient that I sprinkle in now and then with no shame at all.

If you allow yourself to embrace all your feelings and communicate with honesty, then talking about and watching porn can bring tons of joy to sex. Picking out a film together and sharing your reactions to it with one another can be fun and sexy. You might find that you don't get all that far into the scene before you start acting out your own version!

Porn turns a lot of people on, and being turned on is vital for good sex. Watching other people get down and dirty can inspire desire and get your juices going in a major way. You'll need to take the plunge and tell your partner that you want to watch porn with them first though. For all the reasons we have explored, broaching the topic of porn might be a little scary for some. Keep in mind that you don't have to do it perfectly. The conversation can be awkward and funny and still lead to fun and connection. You may wish to do a little research on your own first to find out what porn you like and to make sure it's ethical.

Once you have a sense of what you enjoy, perhaps share a link in an email to your partner with a winky face. Or if you are feeling brave, tell your partner you want a date night at home with the computer. Remember that a lot of people have a strong negative reaction to porn. If you think your partner may feel uncomfortable, start by asking them if they like porn and what their relationship to it is. You can also educate your partner on ethical porn if they are not familiar. Speaking of education, porn can be a great educational tool too.

Sex Ed

Let's be honest, most of us were not educated on how to have sex before we started having it. After all, classes about sexual pleasure, sexual technique, or mindful sex aren't offered in school! We have relied on our own instincts and our partners to lead the way into sexual experience. I had sex for years before I started to really understand how to bring pleasure to myself and others. Porn wasn't as readily available back then, but I've always been passionate about sex. I read books about sex and asked knowledgeable people lots of questions. I think that good porn can also serve as a lesson in good sex.

First of all, watching people being free with their sexuality is a lesson in itself, especially for our sexually-repressed culture. What if seeing a woman have sex with two men was viewed as empowering instead of degrading? If the porn is ethical I find a woman with two men to be a beautiful (and hot) expression of female sexuality and power. Just seeing naked bodies can be educational and freeing for some. It all depends on how you are thinking about it. Let go of the shame; the act is simply human beings in their natural state doing what humans do best.

Watching porn can also help you figure out what turns you on. Maybe you find out that you want to dominate or be dominated by your partner. Maybe you find out that you want to explore something with someone of a new gender. Maybe you just want to dress up in a sexy maid's outfit while you partner watches you scrub the bathroom with a toothbrush. Porn can open your eyes to all new layers of your sexual expression.

You can also pick up some new positions or techniques from watching porn. There are endless ways to have good sex and porn can introduce you to some of them. Keep in mind that some of what you see in porn is more about camera angles than pleasure, so be sure you are placing your focus on pleasure and connection rather than on trying to copy the scene exactly. Also remember that porn performers are professionals. You may not want to try *every-thing* you see in porn at home. For example, one should never put anything in a vagina or mouth that has just been in an anus.

Porn is just one of many things that you can explore in good sex. If it's not your thing, don't worry about it! Always move toward mindfulness and intimacy with yourself and your partner. Even while you are watching an ethical gang bang.

good sex tip

The Rough Stuff

If you are a fan of rough BDSM porn, never fear—that can be ethical too! Be sure to use search terms like "Consensual Non-Consent" and "Ethical BDSM" when looking for ethical porn of this nature. Some of my favorite BDSM content is *The Training of O* series from www.kink.com. These are really intense films that always end with the performer talking to the camera about what a great time they had. This gives the clear message that the performer was totally on board and enjoyed the ride. There is no shame in being turned on by this kind of porn; in fact, many people are. Have fun and always pay for your porn!

Spiritual People Don't Do That!

So, maybe you've read this far and you are thinking, *This chapter is b.s. How can porn be spiritual?* Well, to that I say: *everything* is spiritual. How can anything, porn included, not be spiritual? There isn't some box in the universe where all the nonspiritual stuff belongs. Even if there was, the box would still be a part of this wild, beautiful, and spiritual mystery that our planet is but a small speck of. This isn't to say that watching porn falls within what is right for you. It may not be for you, but if you are experiencing aversion to it because it's not spiritually evolved enough, you may be missing the point of spirituality.

One of the big traps people fall into on the spiritual path is becoming attached to a fixed view of what is spiritual and what is not. This is incredibly limiting. One of the most common ways I see this manifest is through the idea that if you are truly spiritual you always feel good and never, ever get sad or angry. That's why we have a bunch of "spiritual" people who are good at following their breath and saying Namaste but are so bottled up inside that they explode in a fit of fury when someone cuts them off on the freeway. It's also why you see so many spiritual teachers with sex scandals. They are so set on being "spiritual" but don't talk about how they are really feeling; all other human emotions that don't fit the blissed-out-and-compassionate façade get stuffed down. This results in toxic behavior and a lot of suffering. Even if there aren't such obvious negative results like sex scandals, anyone who is repressing real feelings to protect a perfect image is living a disconnected and isolated life.

To live a full and rich life, we must always be willing to peel back the next layer of the onion. We must be willing to investigate our beliefs and preferences. We must be willing to wear our spirituality like a loose garment rather than a corset or straightjacket. We must be willing to wake up again and again without any expectation of graduating to some perfect self. This is of course also true in our sexuality. One thing I've come to understand is that my sexuality is fluid. What turns me on, what kind of lover I'm attracted to, my sex drive, and lots more have changed and changed again over the years. As I've allowed myself to soften into that fluidity, my life has expanded in wonderful ways. If I held tight to my early-twenties version (or early-thirties) of sexuality, I'd be missing out on a lot.

Porn can, understandably, be very triggering for some. It can bring up a very rigid self that is angry, afraid, and judgmental. The same can be said for some folks' reaction to BDSM or certain types of role play, and to celibacy for that matter. That rigid self feels that it needs to defend it's position on what it deems acceptable. It will behoove you to look closely at that self when it comes up due to porn, or anything in life really. Using **FOCUS ON SELF,** you can deconstruct that self and begin to recognize that digging your fingernails into your opinions and preferences is only causing you suffering. This isn't to say that you'll change your mind and want to start watching porn—you may never enjoy it, and that is A-OK. The point is to wake up from the dream that attachment to the self has trapped you in. You can have no interest in porn (or Parcheesi or pickles) but also have no aversion, position on, or judgment of it either. When we come from a place of acceptance we are much more likely to take positive and effective action in reducing suffering in ourselves and others.

Some people have a huge and negative response to the topic of porn. While I'm not saying that you need to like porn to have good sex, I do think that working through aversion will improve your life in many ways and improve your sex life too. Anytime we have strong negative beliefs, about anything, we are limiting our possibility for awakening and of being of service to the world. It is our responsibility to practice acceptance and transmute hatred and judgment into love, or at least neutrality.

I used to have a huge aversion, judgment, and hatred for anyone who sexually abused children. Seems reasonable, right? It's one of the most hurtful and damaging things someone can do to another human. I felt justified in my feelings, and would often say things like, *He should be castrated,* or *She should be put to death,* or *They don't deserve to live.* This mental and emotional experience was painful and caused me to suffer, but I saw no other way to react. After a few years of meditation and some work on my own abuse, I suddenly found that I felt very different. I felt compassion and even love for the people who were in so much pain that they needed to hurt others in such an awful way. I was shocked. All the anger and hatred was gone. I now saw child abusers as more than just that: I saw them as humans.

Thanks to that shift, I am now much more capable of helping people to heal their trauma of sexual abuse. I am more effective, positive, and solution-based. I am a better teacher and I am no longer suffering as a result of my toxic attitude. My new perspective doesn't mean I condone sexual abuse, far from it. I just no longer view those who abuse as nonhuman and undeserving of love or compassion.

As I've said a few times now, I am a porn lover. I don't share this story to compare porn to sexual abuse. I see porn as a fun, sexy, and even healing vehicle. I also don't share this story to pass judgement on how you view abusers. I share this story because it is an extreme example of how we can change when we are willing to look at our beliefs and opinions with clear eyes and an open heart. In this case, most of the work took place under the surface of consciousness. My meditation practice was under the hood giving me a spiritual oil change and I didn't even know it. The side effects of meditation are compassion, unity, and love. Find out for yourself—you have nothing to lose but your own suffering. And, well, on the flip side, the cost of awakening is just everything.

nine

good sex is safe sex

Please note: This chapter explores rape and abortion.

Let's start with this. If you are unable to have the safe sex and sexually transmitted infection (STI) talk with your partners, for any reason, stop being sexually active right now. I'm not joking. This basic level of self-care and sexual mindfulness is mandatory—not just for good sex, but for any sex at all. Anyone who has been diagnosed with an STI or had an unwanted pregnancy will tell you that there is no unprotected sex that feels good enough to make it worth it. There is no reason to contract something, transmit something on to someone else, or need to have an abortion to learn the value of safe sex. Safe sex is easy and it can also be sexy.

If we keep our focus on doing no harm, we are much more likely to get what we want out of a relationship. For some, doing no harm may mean being monogamous, while for others it might mean celebrating your partner's sexual relationships with someone else. You need to get clear on what is authentically right for you and what is right for the relationship. This requires deep self-introspection and the ability to communicate with your partner in a loving and open way. Discussing safe sex and consent at the beginning of a relationship (or before giving your acting class crush a blowjob in the bathroom at a party) sets you up, from the gate, to do no harm.

Because it can be challenging for many folks to discuss safe sex and consent, this can be a place where checking out occurs. Wanting to just get to the good stuff and avoid the uncomfortable sets the stage for crossed boundaries and regrets. To have good and mindful sex, you need to show up for all of it, including the before and after.

I grew up during the AIDS crisis—I knew from a young age that having unsafe sex could have deathly consequences. Even so, it took a few close calls before I really learned to take care of my body during sex. Part of what I had to learn was how to talk about safe sex and sexual histories. By the time I was sixteen, I was skilled in this conversation, and though it was still awkward and uncomfortable to have it, I did anyway. Now I find "the talk" to be fun and even kind of hot. Having that conversation means you are going to be having sex sooner rather than later! It's part of the foreplay. It also means that you love and respect yourself and that the person you are talking to feels the same way about themselves.

Getting Tested

The first step is to go get tested. Get tested for any and all STIs. That way you know where you are starting. If getting tested brings up fear for you, use **FOCUS ON SELF** to deconstruct the fear and **POSITIVITY BOOST** to soothe and comfort yourself. Then, go get tested even if you are still feeling afraid. You can bring a friend and your mindfulness practice with you. Stay in touch with your thoughts and emotions leading up to the testing, during the testing, while you are waiting for the results, and when you receive the results. Tracking your mental and emotional experience will help in keeping anxiety at bay. Here's an STI Test Anxiety Meditation for you.

the practice

- Sit down and relax from your head to your toes.

- Bring to mind the appointment you have coming up. Notice how your body reacts.

- Bring your attention to the area in your body where you are experiencing anxiety. Allow all the resistance to the anxiety to fall away. Soften to the sensation of anxiety.

- Begin to explore the sensation as just a sensation, letting go of the story about the sensation.

- Relax your eyes, jaw, shoulders, and stomach.

- Notice any fluctuations in the sensation you are observing. Keep relaxing around it.

- Try saying the following phrase to the sensation: I accept you just as you are. I love you just as you are.

- When you find yourself pulled into anxious thoughts, just come right back to gently exploring and allowing the sensations in the body.

- Finish with POSITIVITY BOOST. You can continue to work with this exercise leading up to, during, and after the testing while you are awaiting the results.

There can also be a lot of anxiety that comes up while waiting for your results. I've often heard people say that they haven't had any sex at all since their last test, but are still worried while waiting to hear back. This is a perfect example of unnecessary suffering and nonfunctional thinking. If this is happening to you, it's a great opportunity to observe the tyranny of the mind. These thoughts pull you in but can do you no good. The tests have been taken, and you'll get the results. There is no need to think and think and think about it. Notice how your mind says otherwise. You don't have to try to stop those thoughts. Just acknowledge them and then choose to focus elsewhere. You are not those obsessive and pointless thoughts, and you don't have to believe them.

The Talk

Once you have your results, you are ready to have the talk. It is best to talk in person, rather than by phone or text. So much is communicated nonverbally, and trust and intimacy is built through encounters like this. Again, use your meditation in action practice to stay present during this conversation. Remember that it's okay to feel uncomfortable. Discomfort won't kill you.

If either of you has a current STI, it will be a sensitive subject, so be gentle with yourself and your partner. For some, having sex with a person who has an STI is a nonnegotiable no. If you find yourself on either end of that situation, be compassionate and kind to yourself and your partner. For others, this won't be a problem, but discussions about how to protect the uninfected partner will be needed. The good news is having an STI does not mean you will transmit it to your partner. If you take precautions, and special care with any high-risk activities, your partner won't have much to worry about.

Having the talk is a way that you can put mindfulness and self-love into action. You are taking steps to protect yourself and getting to know the person you are about to share your body with. If you attempt to discuss safe sex with someone and they are unable to look you in the eye and engage in an adult conversation, move on. You've dodged a bullet. You deserve a partner who loves themselves and respects you enough to value safe sex. However, it's possible that a potential partner might need support to talk about sex,

---

good sex tip

It's a good idea to hold off on sex until you have both been tested. It's also okay to ask to see the paperwork. If you are just getting to know someone, asking for what you need to build trust is totally reasonable. Getting tested is easy. There are clinics that can give you free, rapid HIV testing, as well as all other STI screenings. I find that these clinics make the process simple and judgment-free. If you are not in need of free testing, make a donation to support those who are. You should get tested once a year, or before you have sex with a new partner. If you are sexually active with multiple partners, it's a good idea to get tested regularly to keep everyone protected.

---

so don't be too quick to judge. If there is willingness to connect and communicate, that means a lot, even if it is uncomfortable.

Once you get past the STI part of the talk, move on to what method of protection you'd like to use. There are tons of options based on what kind of relationship you have. If you are monogamous, protection against STIs may not be necessary at all, but make sure you are both on the same page before putting away the prophylactics.

Knocked Up

I'm at the age when all of my friends are popping out kids, or trying their best to do so. I've only recently started considering the possibility of making a baby. Eighteen years is a long time to be responsible for another human, and from what I hear it's actually a life sentence. Nonetheless, I think I'm almost ready to become a mom. Thanks to practicing mindful and safe sex I get to plan for this big step, rather than have it thrust upon me by a surprise visit from the Stork. This is one darn good reason for having safe sex.

Other than a birth control malfunction, no one should be blindsided by that oversized bird carrying a bundle of joy. Don't kid yourself. You *do* have the power and intelligence to be mindful in your sex life. Not using birth control because *you were in the moment and forgot* is a total cop out. We live in an age where there are many forms of birth control, including the morning after pill.

Everyone makes mistakes, and sometimes (very rarely if used properly) birth control doesn't work. You are then faced with a choice. Making a choice like this will be much less agonizing if you have a mindfulness practice in place. I didn't always have these tools, and I didn't always practice safe sex. There were consequences. Years later, meditation helped me to address and process the choice I made.

Abortion and Healing

When I was twenty, I got pregnant. I had a partner who I was monogamous with, and we often didn't use birth control. I just pushed the thought of unwanted pregnancy to the back of my mind. I didn't have a mindfulness practice at that time, and it was easy for me to lie to myself. Once you start to wake up, you stop being able to be dishonest with yourself for the most part. But at twenty I was fully capable of pulling the wool over my own eyes, and I thought I could get away with not having safe sex.

When I found out I was pregnant, there was no question for me. I would not be bringing this fetus to term. Before I even revealed the news to my partner, I had already made the appointment. I was too early in my pregnancy to get an abortion, so I had to wait. During this time, I pushed down any fears or sadness and tried my best not to think about what was growing inside of me. The last thing I wanted to be was present or mindful with my body. I wanted to pretend that my body didn't exist. Strangely, I didn't drink or smoke while I waited to be able to have the abortion. I knew I wouldn't be having the baby, but I guess I still wanted to protect it in some way.

I cried only twice: very briefly, on the morning of the procedure, and again when I woke up from the anesthesia. But anesthesia always makes me cry. I never actually processed the event or allowed for any grief. I was (and still am) strongly pro-choice, but that doesn't mean that abortion isn't a complicated and sensitive issue for me. At that time, I wasn't capable of confronting the emotions involved with terminating my pregnancy. Ten years later, however, I was ready to take a look at that experience, and I happened to be on a Buddhist meditation retreat.

The first precept in Buddhism (and the sixth Commandment in Christianity) asks followers not to kill. The Buddhist meditation retreats I go to offer only vegetarian meals. Attendees are asked not to kill any spiders or flies they may find in their room, and to be aware of living creatures that may be underfoot. It's not uncommon to see people carefully scooping up a bug that found its way to the middle of a walking path and placing it out of harm's way. I am one of those people. I've never been a fan of killing bugs or anything else.

On this particular meditation retreat, I had been communing with all the creatures of the land. I had become especially fond of the lizards I had been seeing lounging in the sun each afternoon. Toward the last few days of the retreat, I was walking to the building that my room was in, and I nearly tripped trying to avoid stepping on a grasshopper. Suddenly, this thought crossed my mind: *I am going out of my way not to kill a grasshopper, but I killed the beginnings of a human.* I had made the choice to end a possible life. That life could have grown to become my child. This was the first time I had ever considered that truth.

I didn't immediately turn in my pro-choice card or suddenly deeply regret the decision I had made a decade before. I didn't turn on my twenty-year-old self and berate her. Instead, I began to explore the thoughts and emotion that arose as a result of this new perspective.

I spent a lot of time focusing my attention on my stomach and reproductive organs. I gently used my physical awareness to touch into emotions and trauma stored there from the abortion. I felt and heard what my body wanted me to know. I apologized to my uterus for the violation that it had experienced. I communicated with my body in a kind and curious way, listening to all it had to say. I offered myself unconditional love and soothed the sadness that arose.

It was lucky that I was at a retreat when the feeling about the abortion surfaced. I had lots of space to work with it and didn't have to worry about cooking my own meals or going to work. When the abortion came up, I spent a good four hours in meditation, and spoke with one of the teachers at the retreat. She listened with the utmost compassion and then told me that she too had ended a pregnancy in her early twenties. Hearing that from a Buddhist nun was incredibly helpful. She asked if I would do it again, and my answer was (and still is) no, for personal and specific reasons.

We continued to talk and she suggested that I have a ceremony for the child that I chose not to have. When I returned home, I found that a ceremony was healing and offered closure. I lit some candles and spoke to the being that I chose not to bring into the world. Even though I do not regret the choice I made, it was important for me to touch the grief associated with the abortion.

If you have unprocessed feelings about an abortion, yours or your partner's, it can be important to give yourself the time and space to work through them. People often have very polarized feelings about abortions—they are either all bad or all good. That doesn't always reflect the full spectrum of our emotions, however. You can be pro-choice, like me, and still need to grieve an abortion. If you resist your grief because it doesn't go along with your politics, you're not being fully honest with yourself. For some, there may be no grief, and that's okay too. But if you do need to process your experience of having an abortion, your meditation practice can help.

I used a practice similar to this as I was working through my thoughts and feelings about my abortion.

Exploring Past Abortions for Women

Please note: This may be something you want to explore with a teacher or therapist rather than on your own. Partners of women who have had an abortion can use a similar practice to work through this experience as well. Additionally, this is for use only if you have feelings coming up about a past abortion. I don't recommend "digging" up emotions.

the practice

- Have your journal and a pen close by. Sit comfortably, consider using extra cushions to make yourself feel as cozy as possible.

- Relax from your head to your toes.

- Place a hand on your stomach and a hand on your heart and begin by offering yourself these words: I treat myself with love, acceptance, and kindness in all things.

- Now place your attention on your stomach and womb.

- Gently ask this part of your body if there is anything it wants you to know.

- Now notice any thoughts or emotions that arise.

- In a gentle and fluid way, move between the thoughts, both words and images, and the emotional sensations. Pay special attention to any sensations in the area of your reproductive organs and vagina.

- Allow both your body and your mind to communicate with you as you continue to hold a hand on your stomach and on your heart.

- Now write two pages of stream of consciousness writing (SOC). Remember, don't sensor yourself at all.

- After you have written two pages come back to the meditation.

- If any questions or insights arise through the writing you can introduce them in the meditation. Then notice what comes up in response in both the body and the mind.

- Move between the meditation and SOC writing as many times as you like.

- If at anytime you become overwhelmed switch to THE POSITIVITY BOOST.

I didn't have a mindfulness practice when I was twenty. If I had, my guess is that I wouldn't have ever gotten pregnant. I'm sharing this story with you in part to show you how a past abortion can be processed using meditation. I'm also sharing it because this doesn't have to happen to you. If you start being mindful *today* about your safe sex practices, you most likely will not have to face an unwanted pregnancy. Even if you are a strong supporter of the Roe vs. Wade decision, abortion shouldn't be a form of birth control. Just a little bit of mindfulness will help you to put safety first. Accidents do happen, but mindfulness can make that less likely.

Using your method of birth control consistently and responsibly makes the chance of an unwanted pregnancy go down quite a bit. But there's something that comes before condoms, dental dams, or any other safe sex tool. That is consent.

Consent

Having safe sex isn't just about protecting yourself from STIs and pregnancy, it's also about protecting yourself and your partners emotionally and physically. You can do this by practicing radical consent in all your sexual activities. That means saying and hearing *yes* before having sex of any kind. This is another of those non-negotiables in good sex, bad sex, and ugly sex. Consent is required for *all* sex.

When I was a teenager, "No Means No," was a popular anti-rape slogan. But not saying *No* doesn't necessarily mean *Yes*. And saying yes to sex doesn't mean you can't change your mind, and it doesn't mean you are game for anything. Consent is required every time, and for any new sexual adventure.

I was talking with a friend recently about consent, and she said something that hit me to the core. She said, *I was never raped, but there were tons of times I didn't say yes*. That sentence so perfectly encapsulated quite a few of my early sexual experiences. I've heard the same sentiments expressed by many others as well. Learning to ask for and give, or not give, consent is Good Sex 101. Listening for a *Hell Yes,* rather than settling for the absence of a *No*, is a good rule of thumb. "No Means No" is terribly outdated, and is being replaced with "Yes Means Yes," a much more empowering and consent-based phrase.

Consensual sex is when everyone involved says *Yes*. If someone is too drunk to say yes, it's not consensual. If someone is too young to say yes, it's not consensual. If you are in a monogamous relationship and you have sex with someone else, your partner has not consented to that. So, in that way I think of cheating as sex without consent.

Honesty and mindful communication are needed to create clarity on what consent means to you. Bringing mindfulness to your sex life will help you to love yourself enough to say yes when you mean yes, and no when you mean no. It will also help you hear and respect your partner's wishes. As obvious as consent might be to some, for others it's a foreign concept. I didn't understand consent at all when I started having sex. But why would I? I was just a kid.

I Didn't Say Yes

When I was fourteen, I had fallen into a downward spiral of drugs, alcohol, and self-harm. My tumultuous home life had caught up with me, and by age twelve I was already smoking and drinking. In a few short years I had graduated to hard drugs and hallucinogens. I was rarely sober. I kept vodka in a water jug in my closet. I was always looking for a way to check out and drop into oblivion. Age fourteen is also when I started having sex. When I think back to the scrawny, wild child that I was, I just want to send her to rehab and tell her that everything will be okay. But at that age, the best I could do was look for love and attention through sex.

The first guy did ask me for my consent, but the next guy didn't. He was twenty, six important years my senior. We were outside during the early morning hours, in a field, after a party. I was on LSD and had been drinking and smoking pot. I can only imagine that I must have been pretty out of it. I remember saying something about needing a condom, and him saying, *I wouldn't do anything bad to you.* I guess that meant he wouldn't give me an STI, but I'm not exactly sure. Then he had sex with me. I can't remember it at all. I'm sure that I never said, *Hell yes.*

When I see a fourteen-year old girl today and think back on this experience, I shudder. I can't fathom a grown man having sex with the skinny, drunk little teenager that I was back then. I guess he must have been an unhealthy and unhappy person. It wasn't just once either. Since I was drunk or high most of the time, he continued to have sex with an intoxicated kid.

At the time I thought I was *in love*. I would sneak out of the house to see this man and have sex in his truck. Lie and say that I was sleeping over at a friend's house and stay with him. I think this went on for a few months. I know that some family friends tried to end this relationship, but I was a stubborn girl. Once, I even went into a police station to ask if what I was doing was legal. The female cop behind the glass looked at me with concern and asked if I was okay. I mumbled something and ran out.

For the record, I came up positive for the human papilloma virus (HPV) shortly after the relationship ended. I found out that his ex-girlfriend had come down with the same thing prior to him being with me, and he had known. So that added yet another layer to how nonconsensual our sex really was. I was lucky that the strand of HPV I got cleared my system, never to reappear. The one good thing about the STI was that I was forced to learn how to have the safe sex talk at an early age.

So, was I raped? Though it legally was statutory rape, I don't consider myself a rape survivor. But was it *consensual*? No. No. No. It took me many years to understand that, but now it is very clear to me. Not only was he an adult, while I was a child—I was also extremely intoxicated. I was not capable of consenting to sex. I also didn't consent to getting an STD, and my requests for a condom were ignored. This wasn't the only time I had sex without consent. Sadly, it happened many times throughout my teens and early twenties. There were also times when I had sex with someone who was clearly incredibly intoxicated. I'm not proud of that. Part of my making amends to those people is to never do that again with anyone else. Please keep in mind, it is up to each person to decide how they define their sexual experiences. What I don't see as rape for me, you might see as rape for you. I don't mean to define what rape is or is not, only to share my personal experience and perspective.

Today, it's easy for me to only have consensual sex. Consent is a part of my safe sex regimen, which is based in mindfulness and honesty. When I was younger I didn't value myself or my partners enough to truly practice safe sex, including consent. If that's where you find yourself, please put sex on hold and focus on building self-esteem and self-love. Use your meditation practice to explore your feelings about safe sex and consent. You deserve safe, and consensual, sex every single time. We all do.

Talk It Out

Real consent calls for real communication. This is especially true in the beginning of a relationship or during a first encounter. It's better to go a little overboard with consent than skimp on it. I'm not suggesting that you ask and give permission for every move. I am a woman who likes to be kissed without being asked, but only if I've given my energetic consent. That can be a little subtle and requires an attuned and mindful partner. Each situation should be treated separately. With one woman I had sex with recently, I asked for consent every move I made moving toward sex. That felt right. With another woman I didn't need to ask. I could tell from her energy that she wasn't up for anything other than a sweet kiss or two. We need to use our mindfulness to be clear on what is needed with each partner. If you are unsure, I suggest that you always err on the side of too much consent. Remember that saying *I'm not sure, let's hold off on that for now* is a great option if you aren't sure of what you are wanting. There is no rush with sex. It's not urgent, even if your body may think it is. You can take your time to make sure that all parties are fully on board for whatever is going down. Consent can be withdrawn at any time. Consent is fluid just like we are. There may be some aspects of it that don't change much throughout a lifetime and others that change frequently. We are not solid and permanent in any way, including in our sexual tastes and boundaries. This is why it's so important to continue to communicate about what you want and don't want, even when you've been together for years.

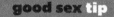

good sex tip

Who says consent can't be sexy? Some good friends of mine created a narrative web series about just how sexy consent can be, called FCK YES.[1] Each episode explores different ways consent can actually be a turn-on. The common thread between all the stories is that clear and honest communication is all it takes to make consent sexy.

Negotiations on consent are not just for new relationships. That conversation continues even after you think you've crossed every possible bridge. This becomes more obvious for those who are in non-monogamous relationships or who explore BDSM. Those rabbit holes can go deep, and become very subtle. I've been on both sides of nonconsensual sex acts with long-term partners. It's not fun, and could have been easily avoided with better communication.

Your mindfulness practice will help you move through challenging conversations with ease. When you are first learning to negotiate sexual boundaries, it's helpful to stay in touch with your body. Keep allowing sensations to arise and pass without tightening up around them. As you learn to accept what is happening in your body, it will find more freedom to say what you need to say. You will also find that your body gives you extremely clear messages about what it does and does not want. **BASIC BODY AWARENESS** and **FOCUS ON EMOTIONS** can be used in action when you are navigating consent.

Meditation is masterful at uncovering the emotions that we have been keeping under the surface. Observing your thoughts with **FOCUS ON MIND** will give you access to deeper layers of your consciousness, and eventually make the unconscious conscious. By practicing meditation every day, you increase the opportunities to wake up to your authentic desires—the first step toward authentic, consensual communication.

Safe Sex Is Self-Love

Getting your consent isn't just your partner's responsibility. Giving someone consent means knowing what you want and then being willing to speak it out loud. I can't tell you how many times I forced myself to have sex when I didn't really want to. I sometimes say that I was my worst abuser. Before I started meditating and healing my past traumas, I treated myself like trash. I didn't even recognize that what happened to me in the field with that older guy was wrong. I had a lot to learn about self-love. I needed to learn to honor myself and my own sexual boundaries. I needed to learn to see and love myself. Part of the work is repairing any broken trust with yourself. When we betray ourselves, especially when sex is involved, we must rebuild trust.

A great way to build trust with yourself in matters of sex is to use the slogan, *Yes Means Yes*. This means only moving forward with a sex act if it's a clear and confident *yes*. If you are feeling even a little unsure if you want to go further, you don't. Even if your partner is superhot. Even if your partner is making it hard to resist.

Even if some parts of you want nothing more than to fuck your partner for hours. It needs to be a full body, full mind, enthusiastic *yes*, before you take that next step. Each time you honor and care for yourself in this way, trust will grow. The same way trust must be earned with a partner, it has to be earned in your relationship with yourself. Treating your body (and your sweetheart) with love by respecting how you really feel will make safe sex a no-brainer.

Protecting yourself from STIs or unwanted pregnancy is an easy way to put self-love into action. If you don't yet have enough self-love to know you deserve to be safe, take a break from sex and put the focus on yourself. By that I mean put the focus on loving yourself. We all know that safe consensual sex is the "right" thing to do, but what makes it right? And why don't we do it?

What makes safe sex and consent right is that it is self-love in action. Self-love is always the right thing to do. The reason you don't always practice safe sex and consent is that on some level you think you don't deserve it. You think you don't deserve it because you haven't cultivated enough self-love to know that *of course* you deserve it.

Your mindfulness practice can show you just how lovable you are. When you choose to sit down and practice meditation, you are loving yourself. Some of that love comes from how good meditation is for you. It lowers your stress levels, helps you sleep better, gives you better concentration and focus, decreases inflammation and so on. Just like eating organic food, meditation is good for you. Meditation also offers love on another level. When you sit with your thoughts, emotions, and aches and pain you make friends with your mind and body. You begin to think more fondly of yourself. You begin to take it a little easier on yourself. You start to fall in love with your beautiful self.

Learning to love yourself (or really your many selves) is a spiritual path all on its own. If you just focused on loving and accepting yourself unconditionally for the rest of your life you'd be a spiritual powerhouse. You would also find that life got easier and easier. It's amazing what someone who has self-love can accomplish. Careers explode, relationships flourish, and good sex abounds.

Every time you have safe sex or have an honest conversation about consent, you are putting self-love into action. Self-love is a state of mind, but it's also a daily practice to bring into your external life. I encourage you to find new ways to love yourself every day.

ten

relax, get to it

Relaxing is a very brave thing to do. Relaxing is a personal revolution. We have tension built up in our bodies for all kinds of reasons—tension that starts to build when we are quite young. As children, we are totally open and vulnerable. We are entirely dependent on our adult (or sometimes pre-adult) guardians to feed us, clothe us, keep our temperature regular, protect us, and love us. Babies are not tense, but by the time we are little kids tension can already be setting in. Our parents, siblings, and relatives pass on their stress and tension to us.

As little ones, we start to form areas of tension in the body, nervous habits, and tics. The tension is there to protect us and to help us brace against the trials of life. Then, we start school and someone makes fun of us or we do poorly on a test, and another layer of tension is added on. When we get a little older, maybe we are in a car accident. We may have no major injuries, but it's enough to add another layer of tension. Then our parents separate, or one of them gets ill or maybe starts drinking too much. Or we find ourselves experiencing a first heartbreak, or a first sexual trauma. By the time we are adults we have knots in our shoulders, headaches, and/or lower back pain. We just can't seem to relax, even on vacation, even when drunk. Our body has learned to be tense, and it thinks it needs to stay that way in order for us to be safe.

Learning to relax means teaching our bodies that they are safe. We have to slowly and gently peel back and dissolve the layers of tension. As we get closer and closer to the original traumas and stresses, the resistance can become even more intense. That's because we are approaching that sweet, innocent self that has been hidden under all the tension for so many years. Our body wants to protect that part of us from ever being hurt again. If we greet that resistance with kindness and patience, it will, day by day, lessen as our body learns to trust us. Eventually, we can start to relate to stresses and traumas in a whole new way. We will let go of these experiences without locking them in. Our bodies don't need to hold all of this tension.

Learning to Relax

I was an incredibly tense child. There are photos of me, as young as five, hunched over, jaw locked, with fingers bloody from all the nail biting. Tension was a big part of my life from very early on. As I got older, the tension piled up. A car accident here, an abusive girlfriend there. By the time I was in my twenties, I was very tightly wound. Relaxing meant making myself susceptible to emotional and perhaps physical danger. When I tried to relax I felt awful. My mind would speed up and I'd get angry or very sad. Drinking and drugs helped, but eventually not even oblivion could soften my edges.

I had daily headaches, back problems, and I would grind my teeth so badly at night that I found shards of tooth in my mouth in the morning. I was a stressed-out gal. When I started to become aware of my suffering through meditation, I didn't immediately recognize how much physical tension I was holding. The first few years of my practice involved a lot of hardcore techniques. I'd meditate for hours without moving, focusing on the most painful and challenging material I could find. I was a bit of an ascetic, using pain to reach deep states of concentration. I pushed through all kinds of discomfort and never practiced relaxation or loving kindness techniques. My spiritual practice was tight and rigid, much like my body.

After a few years of toughing it out, I began to have an inkling that gentle might be better than rough when it came to spiritual practice. Those years of intensity were not without merit. I hurtled along the classical path, encountering insights and awakenings along the way. For me, waking up started out as a series of dramatic crash landings. I'm grateful for the toughie in me who recklessly drove me into awakening, but she takes the back seat these days.

Learning to relax has become a primary purpose in my life. I'm still working on it. I've been training my body to relax in everyday happenings, and when stress or challenging emotions arise. I've found that it is possible to teach the body to automatically relax in situations where it wants to tense up.

One of the first places I noticed the change was in the car. I've had more car accidents than I'd like to recount (some my fault, some not). The trauma of those accidents used to come up a lot when I was the passenger. If the driver hit the brakes a little too hard, or took a turn a bit too fast, my whole body would tighten up, bracing for impact. In reality, being tense actually makes the injuries of a car accident worse, but my body didn't understand that. Once I became aware of this habitual response to my passenger anxiety, I knew I needed to introduce the practice of relaxation. I started intentionally relaxing every time I felt nervous in the car. At first there was a big gap between the tightening up that happened and the introduction of relaxation. But soon the gap became smaller and smaller. One day, I was sitting in the passenger seat, checking out my lip gloss in the side view mirror, and my boyfriend hit the brakes, hard. My body immediately relaxed completely. I had created a new automatic response.

To begin the process of teaching your body to relax, you can practice **REST AND RELAX** daily. Spending even ten minutes a day focused on relaxation will start to encourage your body to relax throughout the day. To enhance your relaxation training, practice **REST AND RELAX** in action as well. While you are sitting at your desk, driving, cooking, having a conversation, reading, or taking a shower, bring some attention to softening and relaxing your body. It will be especially helpful if you practice this while you are engaging with a person or situation that is challenging or stress provoking. If you feel resistance or fear arise, be gentle and kind with yourself. Remember: Relaxing is a brave thing to do.

Relaxed Sex

Sex is supposed to make you feel relaxed, right? There is the quintessential image of someone, naked and sweaty, falling back into a bed with a big sigh, utterly relaxed from a romp in the hay. But while the moment of orgasm may provide a burst of pleasurable relaxation, a lot of folks are not experiencing much relaxation during the act of sex. The reasons vary from worrying about climax, to pain during sex, to insecurity about physical appearance.

From the beginning of my sexual life, I always carried a lot of tension when engaging with a partner. It was part of the way I checked out during sex, locking myself off physically from the other person. It was also simply a habit. I was a stressed-out teenager and adult just like I was a stressed-out kid. I didn't know how to relax—or even that I was so tense.

A lot of my tension during sex involved trying to orgasm. I trained myself to tighten my whole body up in order to reach climax. I couldn't come unless my vagina was under lockdown. I've since talked to many women who have had the same experience, and who believe that extreme tension is required to get off. While some targeted contractions (and releases) can increase pleasure for both men and women, being tense the whole time limits pleasure. It seems to me that when I tightened up and held on, blood was not able to flow as easily, which lessened the pleasurable sensations.

It took practice for me to have relaxed orgasms. For years, I had been relying on tension to make me come. My body would automatically tighten up when I started nearing climax. Releasing tension seemed like letting go of my chance to have an orgasm. I had a lover who once said, "Relax. You've got my cock in a vice grip!" Eventually I began to incorporate more relaxation into sex and got a big surprise. I found that as I learned to relax, my orgasms didn't go away—*they got better*. I had extended orgasms that lasted for what felt like hours. Relaxation led to me having cervical orgasms—also known as deep orgasms. They were more intense than any orgasms I had felt before.

Foreplay and sex become a lot more delicious when you know how to relax. There is a delightful opening that can occur when you let go of tension during sex. Sensations begin to feel more fluid and the breath starts to flow more freely. It might feel like you and your partner can take up more space, spread out, and luxuriate in each other. Sex isn't meant to be bottled up in a tight little ball. Sex is vast, wild, and mysterious. The more we can relax, the deeper we can connect with our partners and the hotter our sex can be. This is taking embodied sex one step further. Once you learn to be aware of your physical self during sex, you can start to relax into your body and access more of what it has to offer you.

You may want to start by exploring relaxed sex with yourself. Like I said, we have tension for all kinds of reasons. It might feel too scary or not enjoyable to relax with a partner at first. I invite you to make a little time for some relaxed self-loving.

the practice

- Start by doing a five-minute REST AND RELAX practice, lying on your bed or another comfy spot.

- Then take a few minutes to breathe deeply and release your pelvic floor muscles. Keep releasing and relaxing in that area as you begin to masturbate.

- You can use the Mindful Masturbation technique, or just do whatever feels good. Your only task is to keep relaxing.

- Notice when you start to tighten up the pelvic floor or any other part of your body. The only muscles that should be working are the ones needed to masturbate.

- Keep relaxing and releasing without judgment.

- Let go of trying to get off and instead relax and breathe.

- If you do have an orgasm, great! If you don't, that's also great! This is about learning to engage sexually without excess tension. Just enjoy the process.

After a little practice with relaxed masturbation, introduce some relaxation into your partner sex. You may wish to do a session of REST AND RELAX before getting things going. Ideally you and your partner could practice together before sex. Encourage relaxation from the start. Relax while you are kissing, touching, and moving into sex. Let your perfectionism go and just do your best to relax as much as possible. You'll be using some muscles, of course, but relax whatever muscles are not in use. You might also want to take turns being physically passive, letting the other partner do all the heavy lifting.

This doesn't have to be all or nothing. If having your focus on relaxation is challenging, you might just do that for some of the lovemaking session, or on and off throughout the session. Good sex is about being flexible with yourself. Being too rigid about relaxed sex can take all the relaxation (and fun) out of it! This doesn't have to be the only way you have sex, but it's important and wonderful to have the option.

Relaxation Fears

Certain questions and insecurities can arise when we consider having relaxed sex. Here are a few.

Isn't my vagina "supposed" to be tight?

No. Your vagina is not *supposed* to be anything. It, just like you, is a living thing that changes and evolves. Learning to relax your vagina will not make it "loose" or limit your partner's pleasure. It will give you more options for how your vagina experiences penetration, which will in turn add variety to your partner's experience. Your vagina is beautiful. It deserves your unconditional love, just like the rest of you.

What about Kegels?

You may have heard of or practiced Kegel exercises (which people with penises can do as well), when you tighten and then release the pelvic floor muscles. Sort of like a pushup for your privates. This can help with increasing pleasure during sex, including giving you stronger orgasms. Kegels also help you to avoid incontinence after childbirth or in old age, and uterine, vaginal, and rectal prolapse. The release in doing Kegels is just as important as the contraction.

If your pelvic floor is especially tight, I would recommend taking it easy on the Kegels and focus on relaxing.

Will I still look hot if I'm relaxed?
Shouldn't I be flexing and sucking in?

You are hot just the way you are. And learning to relax during sex and otherwise will probably make you look and feel younger. Good sex means loving and cherishing your body. Part of caring for your body includes feeding it healthy food and giving it exercise. It also includes letting it enjoy sex without being shamed or judged. If how you look during sex is keeping you from being able to relax, practice the self-love exercise discussed earlier in the book. Send love to your body, even the cellulite and flab. Do that for a month every day and see how your love for your body blossoms.

What if I get so relaxed that I cry during sex?

I'd say that's a good sign. It means you've allowed yourself to open up deeply. It's normal to be overwhelmed with emotion during or after sex. A loving and mindful partner will have no problem with you crying—in fact, they may recognize that it means they did something right.

Just Breathe

There are two things that many people don't do enough of. One is relaxing, and the other is breathing. How often are you running around, doing your day-to-day tasks, full of tension and taking only shallow breaths? The answer for most folks is *most of the time*. Bringing a little mindfulness to your muscular and cardiovascular systems will bump your quality of life way up.

Let's do some breathing and relaxing right now. I call this Relax and Reset.

---

the practice

- Sit comfortably and take a deep, intentional breath through your nose.

- Feel the breath fill you up from your stomach to your upper lungs.

- Pause briefly at the top of the breath.

- Now, exhale all the breath through your mouth with a sigh.

- As you exhale, let your whole body relax. Release your shoulders and your jaw. Let it all go.

- Feel the relaxation in your body.

- Do this two more times, filling up with more breath on each inhale and relaxing more with each exhale.

How do you feel? I'm going to bet you feel more relaxed than you did a minute ago. This is an exercise you can do many times throughout the day, and I suggest that you do. It's a great way to infuse your day with relaxation and to encourage deep breathing.

Breathing fully is something that a lot of people are not doing on a regular basis. Have you noticed how often you actually take a nice deep breath? In yoga class a few times a week, maybe? Shallow breathing, or actually holding the breath, seems to be a chronic issue for a lot of people.

---

good sex tip

Not sure how to relax your pelvic floor? Let's start with finding your pelvic floor muscles. They are a web of muscles and tissues that surround the anus and genitals. You can feel them easily if you stop peeing midstream and then start again. It's your pelvic floor muscles that are starting and stopping the flow. People with vaginas can relax their pelvic floor by focusing on their vagina and intentionally relaxing the area. People with penises should bring attention to the anus and butt and then relax. You can use BASIC BODY AWARENESS to bring your attention to the genitals, and then direct some REST AND RELAX to the area.

Learning to Breathe

In my late twenties, I was introduced to an actor's voice training technique called the Fitzmaurice Technique, which is all about breathing and relaxing. My teacher, Saul Kotzubei, led me through exercises that gave me deep access to my breath and profound states of relaxation. It was a big insight for me to realize how little I was actually breathing most of the time. After a workshop with him I felt like my lungs had actually gotten bigger. Really, I was just breathing more fully. I am still learning to consistently allow myself to fully breathe, but there has been a massive improvement. Doing exercises like REST AND RELAX, going to yoga, and continuing with voice classes and breathwork is quite helpful. The more I encourage breath and relaxation in my life, the more enjoyable my life is.

I remember when I first discovered the intense pleasure of breathing deeply during sex. I had a friend visiting from Florida, and she had recently been exploring ecstatic breathing techniques. She shared with me how breathing deeply during sex intensified her orgasms tenfold. She explained how the breath moved the pleasure through her body in waves. I was keen to experience these oceanic orgasms for myself, and tried it the next chance I got. My friend hadn't been exaggerating. It was divine.

Here's a simple breathing exercise you can practice with your partner. You can also do it on your own while masturbating.

—

the practice

- During foreplay, start taking deep, full breaths and encourage your body to relax.

- Ideally, you and your partner will be breathing in unison.

- Soften into the sensations you are experiencing.

- Breathe deeply, all the way down to your pelvic area.

- Relax.

- As you start to move into penetration or any other sex act, continue to relax.

- With each in breath, invite the pelvic floor to expand and relax.

- With each out breath, contract the pelvic floor, drawing it upward.

- Then, with the in breath, relax that area even more.

- Continue this breathing throughout the session.

You may find that you have some strong emotional openings while you practice this breathing exercise. Deep knots inside of you can untangle as you release tension and allow your body to fully experience the breath. Let the emotions, as well as any jerks or twitches in your body, arise and pass while you continue to breathe and relax.

Learning to invite breath into sex is a necessary ingredient for good sex. Once you feel it you'll know just what I mean. Breathing and sex are the best of bedfellows. Add relaxation to the mix, and we are getting into some Tantric sex territory.

Tantric Lovin'

Tantric sex has been around for over 5,000 years. It has truly stood the test of time. In Tantric sex, the lovers weave and expand the flow of energy between them through breath, eye contact, relaxation, and other sexual practices. This creates more intimacy and connection, as well as otherworldly pleasure. Exploring Tantric sex is a great option for many who are looking to improve their sex lives. There is, however, often dogma and firm philosophy within this tradition. If that isn't your jam, not to worry. You can borrow from the practice of Tantric sex without buying the cow.

Two of the main themes in Tantric sex are breath and relaxation. Tantra takes the emphasis off of orgasm and puts it on deep connection and spiritual merging with your partner. Some of the practices of Tantric sex involve relaxing and breathing with your partner, while moving very slowly or not at all. This is almost entirely the opposite of how most people are having sex. Most people think of sex as hard and fast. While fucking can be absolutely delightful, it's nice to have other options too. Tantric sex is a very special kind of lovemaking, and it can take time to develop a taste for it.

In our incredibly fast-paced world, slowing down for anything can be a challenge. We have everything the Internet has to offer at our fingertips, we have multi-hyphenate careers, and an app for *everything*. Everyone seems to be racing the clock to catch some imagined goal—the thing that will make us feel complete. It's no wonder so many people are chronically stressed-out and exhausted. The antidote for this fatigue is simply slowing down, breathing, and relaxing. Learning to make love slowly and with relaxation is something that can expand our sexual awareness and teach us to take it a little easier in general. Sexuality is a spiritual path—that's what Tantric sex teaches us. Tantra values relaxation and breath as a primary component of good sex. It gets more complicated than that, but those are some basic tenets. I don't personally subscribe to one right way of having sex, so I take what I like and leave the rest when it comes to Tantric sexual practices. I do, however, think that Tantra can offer invaluable guidance in the realm of breath and relaxation.

Here is an exercise based on Tantric sex practices.

the practice

- Lie naked, face to face with your partner, without touching.

- Make and sustain eye contact. If you are too close to see each other's eyes, move back a bit.

- As you gaze into your partner's eyes, bring attention to the movement of sensations inside your own body.

- Pay special attention to the movement and change, the flow, of the sensations. Take some time with this.

- Slowly, when your bodies are ready, begin to softly and slowly touch your partner.

- Allow the sexual energy between you to build as you explore your partner's body.

- Move slowly. If you think you are moving too slow, move two times slower.

- You can keep your eyes open or close them.

- As you begin to make love keep the pace very slow.

- If you have a penis, don't worry about staying hard.

- Let this experience be fluid. Don't have an aim of orgasm. Don't have an aim at all. Let your bodies and the energy between them move and flow.

- If you are having penetrative sex, don't thrust fast and hard. Instead, ever so slowly move together. Find moments of not moving at all.

- Find the pleasures that are hidden inside, usually masked by the more obvious sensations of sex.

- When you are done, make sure to take some time to hold each other and verbally process the experience.

Slowing down and not "performing" during sex can bring insecurities and attachment to the forefront of consciousness. There can be a lot of identity wrapped up in how you have sex, and trying something new can be confronting. We like to stick with what we are good at. Slowing down will reveal aspects of yourself that you may have been hiding behind your ability to fuck with abandon. Now you have to actually be with your partner, in a soft stillness, stripped down to a bare and profound connection. As you uncover the insecurities and attachments and let them peel away, you'll find an entirely new way of relating to yourself and your partner. You'll have a new wrench in your sexual tool kit.

Relaxing into Pain

Being mindful means taking the time to actually have the experience you are having. I used to be chronically busy, speeding through life. I never stopped to smell the roses. There were too many things to get done! My sex life was a reprieve from my busy life, but I didn't suddenly become mindful while having sex. This made it difficult for me to really listen to what my body wanted during sex. If my body didn't like something, I tended to just push through it, ignoring pain or discomfort.

For people who experience pain during sex, relaxation can be a lifesaver. For most, there is a tendency to tighten up and brace against pain. I used to just clench my jaw, tighten my vagina, and squeeze my eyes shut when I experienced sexual pain. On some level I believed that sex was supposed to be painful some of the time. I've come to know that sex should only be painful if you want it to be (and have a safe word!).

(Note: If you are having pain during sex it could be a sign of a health issue and it's always a good idea to talk to your doctor. Mindfulness is great, but sometimes Western medicine is required.) If you are enduring sexual pain and thinking that it's just supposed to be this way, think again. You deserve to feel good. Recognizing that you are tolerating unnecessary pain is an insight worth exploring. Perhaps there are other areas of life in which you are toughing it out and don't need to be. Many people have deeply embedded beliefs that they deserve to be in pain. You can work through these old belief patterns using **FOCUS ON SELF** to deconstruct the thoughts and emotions involved. Remember to also offer yourself lots of love, patience, and acceptance during this process. It's also good to work with a therapist or meditation teacher on this kind of material.

It's always important to tell your partner if you are experiencing unwanted pain. If you've been open and honest about the pain and want to try to work through it, you can use relaxation and breath to help you. Make whatever adjustments in position, penetration depth, and speed you need to be as comfortable as possible. Don't push through intense pain. Be gentle with your body. Here is an exercise to help you relax and breathe into pain, rather than brace against it.

—

the practice

- Before having sex, set the intention with your partner to practice this technique.

- Use deep breathing and relaxation from the beginning of the sex session.

- When you start to experience pain, let your partner know. At that point, back off of whatever is hurting and find stillness.

- Take a few breaths and relax.

- Very slowly begin to move closer to the point of discomfort.

- Very gently move into a small amount of discomfort. Then breathe fully, directing breath to the pain. Relax all around the pain. Pause there, breathing and relaxing until the pain subsides.

- If it continues to hurt or becomes more painful, back off and then try again.

- If the pain does subside, you can move a little deeper and continue the exercise.

- Always go slow and pause as needed. Work toward letting go of all tension and breathing into any discomfort.

> ## good sex tip
>
> For people experiencing pain during sex, receiving pelvic floor massage can help. Here's what Kimberly Ann Johnson, author of *The Fourth Trimester,* has to say about it:
>
> Pelvic floor massage is a way to directly contact the territory that is painful in a respectful and gradual way so that the people can come into contact with the territory on their own terms. Uncoupling the genitals with pain is a crucial step for any person stepping into their erotic potential and self-empowerment. Getting massage on a part of the body that is usually considered separate, that is conspicuously avoided and draped meticulously, is part of the awakening. Deciding that this part of our body deserves loving attention and touch too, and that that can happen outside of a medical scenario or a lovership scenario is a step in maturity and healing in and of itself. Mindful touch can help people re-associate with areas that may have either experienced trauma or be storing trauma. With re-association often comes a resurgence of authentic desires.[1]

I have had several sessions of pelvic floor massage with great results. I was suffering from chronic inflammation of the bladder and urinary tract and experienced relief after the massage. It also seemed to give my sex drive a boost!

Grasping and Acceptance

Grasping is another word for holding on too tightly to something. Do you find yourself grasping on to pleasure during sex? Well, you're not alone. A big portion of grasping during sex is related to reaching climax or holding off on climax. New students often report feeling all tied up inside in anticipation of orgasm, becoming tense, and narrowing their attention to that one goal. This sexual grasping can be a manifestation of grasping in other parts of life. I know that I used to always be afraid that I wouldn't get what I wanted or would lose what I had. This attitude makes for a very small life. Trust me, I know.

The mind is built to grasp, and then inevitably distorts what it grasps. The more it grasps, the more it distorts. This cycle leads to suffering. It's not just our minds that grasp and distort. Our bodies can do the same thing. The more tension, or grasping, we have in the body, the more distorted our relationship with the body becomes. With more tension comes more pain, and more reason to avoid embodiment. As you learn to relax your body, the grasping will lessen. This will in turn lower the grasping in the mind, leading to less and less needless suffering. Training your body to relax during sex will translate over into the rest of your life. The pleasure you get from relaxed sex will give your mind and body the message that grasping is for the birds. As you fully see how much you are grasping, you'll start to see the path out of grasping and into acceptance.

When I'm in the company of someone who is deeply awake, their level of relaxation is palpable. It's a physical, mental, emotional, and spiritual relaxation that infuses all of their actions, even the subtlest of movements. My experiences with relaxation of this kind have been a roadmap for my own awakenings. This type of relaxation comes when you truly give in to each unfolding moment, without judgment or expectation. Even tiny flashes of this kind of relaxation can be utterly transformative. You can relax your way to good sex, and perhaps into radical acceptance.

eleven

can't get no satisfaction

Many people in long-term relationships report either not wanting as much sex as their partners, or wanting more. Some couples aren't having sex at all because of that disconnect. Mindfulness can help us move through a low sex drive and into an even deeper sexual connection than we had in the early days of a relationship.

A meditation practice makes it hard to hide from your feelings. If you are feeling sexually disconnected from yourself and/or your partner, you'll know it. That awareness is already a step toward reinvigorating your sexuality. It's your job to keep shining that light of awareness on your sex life.

Mindfulness will also help you to understand the reasons behind your or your partner's low sex drive. Being mindful with challenging experiences leads to acceptance. Acceptance of what is happening in the moment allows you to be kinder and more patient with yourself and others. This kindness and patience will be required to move through times when sexual connection is hard to come by.

Not Getting Lucky

Years ago, I had a string of relationships with people who were not interested in having sex with me. In the beginning we had tons of sex, of all kinds, and with abandon. But after a while the sex dwindled down to almost nothing. Before I had a daily meditation practice, I didn't handle this well. I would cry, fight, and lie in bed next to my partner, sulking. I would agonize over what I wasn't getting, and how we needed to fix the problem. I took their low sex drive as a personal insult. What I didn't know at the time was that not getting laid was triggering a deep wound in me.

For many reasons, I equated sex with love. If my partner didn't want to have sex with me, I subconsciously believed that they didn't love me. Before meditation, I didn't recognize what was happening. All I knew was that I felt awful, abandoned, and hopeless. I would cry and complain without taking the time to really look into what was going on. My reaction, of course, didn't elicit a positive response. It made the divide between my partners and myself even greater.

When I introduced a daily meditation practice into my life, I started to wake up to the subconscious workings of my mind and emotions. I also began to see that in every problem there was a path to a deeper awakening. So I set out to utilize my new insight in my discomfort with being denied sex.

Over time, I learned to allow and accept my feelings of frustration. At first, I would need to get out of bed and go meditate in the bathroom until I felt less overwhelmed. Then I was able to stay in bed and continue interacting in a kind way with my partner. I was able to let the disappointment of not having sex pass through me. This made the experience less personal and less painful. As I became more advanced in my practice, I uncovered the self that felt it needed sex to be worthy of love. As soon I saw this as only a story, and not *true*, that self vanished.

All of this is not to say that you should stay in a relationship that doesn't meet your needs. Your partner will need to meet you halfway and work on their side of the issue. I don't recommend resigning yourself to a sexless relationship, or secretly getting sex elsewhere. If you have done all you can do to address the situation and your partner isn't willing to budge, it may be time to move on. At the same time, be gentle, compassionate, and kind as you discover if this is the right relationship for you. For some, low sex drive or sexual blocks can be the result of past sexual abuse. Even if that's not the case, this material doesn't get worked out overnight. It will take time and perhaps professional assistance.

Mindfulness alone may not be enough to shift your sexual connection with your partner. There are many types of sex therapy or coaching that can help with this issue. Get all the support you can. It will be worth it.

Make the most of this time. If you are not getting the sexual connection you desire, use the challenge as an opportunity to grow. Start focusing on what desire and unrequited sexual energy has to teach you. An important part of the spiritual path is learning to observe our desires with equanimity.

Deconstructing Desire

There is nothing wrong with desire. We all experience desire every-day: We desire to eat when hungry, drink when thirsty, and sleep when tired. Sexual desire is like that—simply a human desire. How you react to your sexual desire is the difference between it becoming a vehicle for suffering or something that you can learn from.

All desire is made up of the same stuff: our thoughts and emotional sensations. **FOCUS ON SELF** can show you desire is no different from any other manifestation of self. You can work with it the same way you would sadness, anger, joy, or embarrassment. Once you learn to deconstruct desire in one area, it will be easier to deconstruct other desires as well.

Try the following exercise with something less challenging than sexual desire first, such as food, to get a taste for how it works.

—

the practice

- Buy a food that you love. Wait until you really want it, perhaps before lunchtime, so that the desire level is high.

- Set up the food at your table and sit down.

- Look at the food. Smell the food. Don't eat the food.

- Start to explore the thoughts and emotional sensations that arise. Separate the emotional sensations from the purely physical sensations of hunger.

- If you can't do that, simply observe all sensations along with thoughts.

- Notice any pleasurable sensations of desire that arise.

- You can keep your eyes open or close them.

- Keep greeting the experience of desire for the food with mindful acceptance.

- Notice how desire comes in waves. It's not a static thing, it's moving and changing, sometimes vanishing completely.

- Meditate through at least three waves of desire before eating the food.

- When you do eat it, stay with the pleasurable sensations that flood your body.

- Enjoy the satisfaction of that desire. And then let it go.

Now, try something similar with your sexual desire. You can even do this in bed next to your partner. It's a hell of a lot better than sulking, complaining, and blaming. Get to the bottom of your desire so that you will be better able to mindfully find a solution for the lack of sex in your relationship.

Cultivating acceptance with sexual desire doesn't mean trying to scrub yourself clean of all wanting. Like I said, there is nothing wrong with desire, including sexual desire. Unless you plan to spend some time being celibate, these suggestions are not meant to rid you of the wonderful feeling of wanting to fuck or make love. Instead, this work will help you not to be overrun and overwhelmed with desire. When you are contracted around wanting, and suffering as a result, it's hard to connect with your partner or enact positive change.

Not in the Mood

I went through a period of low sex drive while I was in the process of preparing to write this book. This was strange and uncommon for me, and the fact that I was writing about the joys and wonders of sex at the time made it all the odder. I was the woman who loved sex and could never get enough. Where had she gone? She wasn't as solid as I wanted to think she was. Honestly, I knew she wasn't permanent, but I hated to see her go. It was fun inhabiting that self.

Meditation can show us that there is no solid self that we can rely on to stay the same. Instead, we learn that there are endless arising's of self. These selves are made up of thoughts and emotional sensations. That's it. Most people are walking around with total belief that they are their thoughts and emotions. In doing so, they limit themselves to a very small version of who they can be.

You are NOT your thoughts and emotions. Yes, your thoughts and emotions are part of what makes up your experience, but that's not all you are. You don't have to believe everything your thoughts and emotions express. And you certainly don't have to act on them. It's okay to witness the activity of self in meditation. You don't have to get involved. This saying can be helpful: Don't just do something. Sit there.

One of the many downsides of believing your thoughts and emotions to be you is that you become very attached to certain versions of yourself. All the energy that goes into holding on to who we think we are could be better used finding out what we actually are: something vast, without edges, and beautifully mysterious. When my hypersexual self was ready to die, I mourned but did not hang on to her sleeve and beg her to stay. I knew that this was the next natural evolution in my spiritual development.

I'm what Buddhists call a "householder." I don't live in a monastery, and I have a career, rent to pay, and a romantic partner. It was important to me to continue to nurture my relationship. Part of that meant working through my low sex drive and finding a new way to connect sexually. My partner was incredibly supportive and understanding, and also challenged at times. It's a bummer to get turned down again and again, as I well knew based on my past experiences. I was pretty sure that my sex drive would return at some point, I just didn't know when.

I knew I couldn't rush the process that was unfolding. The transition from who I had been sexually to who I would become was going to take as long as it took. What I could do was be patient and kind with myself as the evolution occurred. I could also take some action. Because I had experience coaching others through low sex drive issues, my tool kit was full.

The Sex Drive Boost Tool Kit

Your sexuality is a relationship like any other. It needs your attention and care. Often times, especially in long-term relationships, people stop nurturing their own sexuality and then wonder why they never have sex.

I suggest that you attend to your sexuality the same way you would with your spiritual practice, physical exercise, or a relationship with a dear friend. Give it time, attention, commitment, and mindfulness. Don't just expect it to dole out benefits without any effort on your part. Good sex requires that everyone involved has a healthy and active relationship with their own sexuality. Engaging with yourself in this way will make you available to support and nourish your sexual relationship with your partner.

Just like any part of your life, your sex life needs your energy. There may be times when most of the energy needs to go elsewhere, but don't forget to feed your sexual piggybank a bit every day. Give at least a little attention to the sexual health of your relationship even when your schedule is full. There are lots of small ways you can do this. The tools that I've included here are only a few that have been helpful to me and others. You'll need to tailor your tool kit to best suit you and your partner's needs.

With all of these tools, I invite you to use your mindfulness practice as you try them out. Notice how your body feels as you learn new ways to connect with your partner sexually. Stay in touch with the activity of thoughts and emotions, and remember you don't have to attach yourself to any one identity. Always work toward what in Buddhism is called the Middle Way: the middle point between excess and denial. Don't become attached to outcomes or getting it right, but don't hold back and limit your expansion either. Balance is the aim here.

Texting

Text messaging is a fun and simple way to create and sustain sexual energy with your partner. It's a kind of daily foreplay practice right at your fingertips. A sexual text can be anything from a sweet and suggestive text to an X-rated video message you make on your lunch break. Even just a few sexy texts a day could help you to relight that spark. This is also a great thing to do while in a long distance relationship or when you are away from your partner for extended periods. Skype and other kinds of video chat can also come in handy when you are apart and wanting to keep your sexual connection alive.

Remember that tone is often lost in texting. You might mean one thing, and your partner might read something very different. Your mindfulness practice will help you to navigate any misunderstanding, but sometimes you need to put down the device and just talk in person.

The Sensual Life

Adding more sensuality to your life can easily translate into more sex. Buy some new bedding in warm and fiery red tones. Wear silk. Make a meal that turns you on. Light delicious and earthy-scented candles. Create a playlist of rich and sensual music. Repaint your bedroom. Try a new perfume or cologne. Enjoy the sensations of your breath.

Directing your attention to sensuality and refining your aesthetic tastes in creative ways will awaken those parts of you. As you sink into beauty and your sensual nature, allow the ripples to reach your sexual expression as well.

Dress for Success

The way we feel on the inside is often reflected in how we present ourselves outwardly. If you are in the midst of a drop in your sex drive, you might find that working from the outside in can help. Give yourself a little extra time to get ready each morning, even if you work from home. Take your time bathing and grooming. If you wear makeup, apply it gently and with mindfulness. Style your hair the way that you find most flattering. Choose the clothing that you feel most attractive in. Starting your day in this way will give you a sense of self-love that can ignite some sexual energy inside of you.

This is all about how you feel, not what others think. If overalls and a bonnet make you feel attractive, go for it!

Pleasure Abounds

There are so many pleasurable experiences in any given day, and learning to tune into them can enliven your sexual self. Eating, urinating, and lying down at the end of the day are all simple activities that can actually be quite pleasurable. All it takes is your attention to change these activities from routine to profoundly pleasure producing.

Sensitizing yourself to pleasure will open you to receive more. Simple pleasure awareness can jumpstart your sex drive by reminding you how good it feels to feel good. Remember that truly enjoying pleasure requires letting go of attachment to pleasure, untangling from thoughts, and being in your body. The **PLEASURE BOOST** can help you to notice and explore pleasure and have equanimity toward it.

Take the Pressure Off

When one is on either side of a period of low sex drive, there can be a lot of pressure. Every night as you climb into bed there is both a sense of doom and a distant hope. The longer you go without having sex, the more the pressure builds. A movie with a sex scene reminds you that you are not having sex. Your newly partnered friends who are in the first flush remind you that you are not having sex. It starts to feel like there's nothing that doesn't remind you that you are not having sex! This pressure can begin to put the relationship in a frozen state. All the fun drains out, and there is a sense of disconnection. What you need is to get connected in a fun way.

Something I sometimes suggest at this juncture is to take sex off the table. For the low-sex drive partner, this can be a huge relief. For the partner with higher sexual desire, this can actually be a relief as well—if sex is off the table, you can relax and not worry about being rejected. But when you take sex off the table, you have to replace it with something fun.

First, set a period of time to take sex off the table. I suggest two weeks. During this time, I highly recommend connecting physically with each other. Cuddle, hold hands, even make out, but take any version of sex out of the scenario. You may find that when the pressure of sex is no longer there, affection comes easier and more often. The low sex-drive partner isn't worried that they will disappoint when a spooning session doesn't turn into sex. The partner with a higher sex drive doesn't have to worry about feeling rejected. Sit down with your partner and write a list of fun activities you can do together for the two-week period. Aim to have at least a few big-ticket items. Maybe a weekend trip to the desert or the mountains, skydiving, or a trip to the theater. If money is an issue, Google cheap and free things to do in your city. There are lots of options. Along with the more ambitious activities, plan a bunch of simple and fun outings or homebound activities. Do a puzzle together, learn to play chess, go on a hike that you've never done before, try a dance class, read a funny book aloud, have a dance party in your living room, binge watch a silly show, and eat take out for lunch and dinner. You get the idea.

If you truly commit yourselves to this endeavor, you will be delighted with the results. You'll feel closer and the relationship will be energized with all the fun you've had. This is a version of the **POSITIVITY BOOST** in action. Rather than directing your attention to what isn't feeling good, you instead focus on what does.

After the period of no sex, plan a time to reintroduce it. Give yourselves a few hours to hang out in your birthday suits. Take your time and keep coming back to relaxation and breath. It is a good idea to keep the expectations neutral. You may not have sex that first time or even the second. But if you can move through whatever happens with a fun and loving attitude, you'll be headed down the right path.

The Bases

When I was a kid there was a lot of talk about the bases. First base was kissing. Second base was hands under the shirt, and shirt off. Third base was hands down the pants, and pants off. A home run was pretty self-explanatory. For the purposes of this exercise, let's include any oral sex in the home-run category. Using these bases can be a fun and low-pressure way to connect sexually.

Set a "First Base Date." You can include dinner and movie, or it can be a time purely reserved for kissing. Try to recall and encourage that feeling of a first kiss. Explore each other's mouths. Kiss until your lips are swollen. But don't go past first base. Set your next date to go to second. Next, set a date for third base. Plan a little extra time for this one. First through third is a lot of territory to cover if you are taking your time. Finally, set the date for a home run. Don't forget the other bases on your way there!

Use your mindfulness practice as you have fun working your way through the bases. **BASIC BODY AWARENESS** and **PLEASURE BOOST** are two techniques that will help you stay with your body and focus on all the delightful sensations.

good sex **tip**

There are few things that are better or more arousing than an amazing kiss. It's an important part of a sexual relationship, and deserves to be talked about. You might start the conversation by asking what your partner likes best about kissing. From there, see where the conversation goes—you both might learn something about each other's preferences and turn-ons.

When doing this exercise, remember that you can always stop. You can always go back a base. Consent is always a rule in this game.

A Little More Talk, A Little Less Action

I dedicated a whole chapter to communication because of how important it is. I want to revisit that now. More often than not, I hear about couples not having sex because one or both of them are not getting what they want. For example, I've heard from many women that they want their partner to be more aggressive and dominant. I also hear from people that they want slower lovemaking, more foreplay (use those bases!), certain toys or props to be involved or to incorporate porn into sex with their partners. Because so many people are too shy to talk about sex, their desires are never spoken aloud. So, rather than open up and speak, they just opt to limit sexual contact. That is a real shame.

In our culture, sex is still taboo, and people don't know how to talk about it—not even with their partners. I suggest that you start your own sexual revolution by asking for what you want. You can be scared, but do it anyway. You can be embarrassed, but do it anyway. The more you express your sexual wants and needs, the more comfortable you will get with it. If you have a partner that isn't willing to answer your call, you may need to reexamine the relationship. If they don't want what you want, it doesn't make them wrong or bad. But it might make them not the right person for you. You won't know until you ask.

Kindness, patience, and compassion for yourself and your partner are the keys to good communication. Allow those traits to be the foundation for asking for what you want and discussing what your partner wants. If one of you is unable to be present and mindful, take a breather and come back to the talk when you can both hold space for each other.

Awakened Role-Playing

What eventually turned out to be most helpful for me in reconnecting with my sex drive was role-playing. No, not that kind of role-playing. There were no sexy nurse outfits, or badly done accents. What I'm referring to is a lot simpler and doesn't involve any props. It just requires you, and the awareness that there is not only one you.

On any given day, endless versions of self arise and pass. There's the you who wakes up grumpy, or the you who wakes up feeling refreshed. There's the you who is annoyed that your partner forgot to buy toothpaste, and the you who wants poached eggs today. There is the you who flirts with the cutie in the elevator, and the you who is feeling the pressure of an upcoming deadline. There is the you who feels a pang of grief when thinking about your orange striped cat that died a few months ago, and the you who enjoys the scent of a black Sharpie pen. All of these selves are made up of thoughts and emotions—impermanent material. There are never-ending selves, and when you fully understand that, you can begin to choose which self you want to inhabit moment by moment.

This freedom to be who you want to be is a fantastic tool for increasing your sex drive. This is an advanced practice and may not be available to everyone. As you continue to dive into your mindfulness practice, it will start to make more sense. Here is an example of how you might engage in awakened role-playing.

---

the practice

- Relax from your head to your toes.

- Begin to observe the activity of the mind and emotions using **FOCUS ON SELF.**

- Notice how every thought and every sensation appear and then vanish. None are permanent. Acknowledge this.

- Become aware of how even the self that is doing the acknowledging is impermanent.

- Now, begin to generate thoughts of your sexual self. These can be images or words. The thoughts can be of you in positive sexual situations, or other images and words that create arousal.

- Notice the sensations of sexual arousal in your body.

- Play around with different versions of your sexual self. The you that likes to make sweet and gentle love. The you that enjoys to be dominated or to dominate your partner.

- Inhabit these versions of yourself fully and without any judgment.

- Become these selves as a great actor becomes the character.

Having low sex drive or a partner with low sex drive can seem like a big problem. Actually, like any other "problem," this challenge can make way for gifts you never expected. Low sex drive can lead you to new ways of making love, more honest communication, and even new ways to explore awakening.

A Pitch for Celibacy

Taking some time off from sex (even with yourself) can be a powerful way to grow emotionally, sexually, and spiritually. If you find yourself in dysfunctional romantic relationship patterns, taking sex out of the equation can help tremendously in creating a shift. Sometimes abstinence can also be vital for healing when working through sexual trauma. There are also some who decide that sex, and everything that comes with it, is an unnecessary distraction from waking up. Many monastic traditions have adopted a vow of abstinence as a way to more fully focus on the path of spiritual awakening. You can probably guess that I won't be taking that route anytime soon.

Around the time that I quit drinking and set my sights on waking up, I decided to take six months off from sex. I had been in one disastrous relationship after another, and I was ready for a new experience. It was suggested to me that I shouldn't date or have sex for a while, and with much hemming and hawing, I begrudgingly took the challenge. I can't say I did it perfectly, but I did my best. A few months in, I had one little almost slip with an ex-girlfriend that ended in me crying. That made it clear that I needed to stay on the abstinence wagon. After six months, I tried again, with awkward consequences. This time it was a handsome guy with good tattoos who was an amazing kisser. That also didn't go so well and we didn't hit a home run. I felt sad, confused, and just not ready. I decided to tack another six months onto my abstinence.

At the end of my year of celibacy, I found myself two weeks into a relationship with an incredibly kind man. On Valentine's Day we said *I love you* for the first time and had sex. Yep, kind of sickeningly sweet, but it was lovely. It was probably some of the most connected and intimate sex I had ever had up until that point. That relationship was my first fairly healthy one. No cheating, no lying, and no abuse. That was the beginning of me finding out that it was possible to have a loving and functional romantic relationship. I know that the year of celibacy was a major factor in that change.

When I go on meditation retreats or do certain spiritual practices, I abstain from sex for set periods of time. It's always quite easy to do, perhaps because I have completed that year of abstinence. I actually quite enjoy those periods. It's a time for me to delve into other parts of myself and direct my focus in a sharp and clear way. I certainly suggest trying this out, even for just a few weeks. If you have a partner, you'll have to negotiate with them on this. Don't forget that you and your personal growth are not the only thing that matter when you have a honey. If you want to live like a monk long term, you might need to let your lover go, or find one who wants to be celibate too.

You can use your meditation tools to address any cravings or strong emotions that arise during your sex-free time. There is a lot of fuel for your psycho-spiritual growth available when you remove such a primal activity from your life. Use it!

I remember the first time I noticed how mindfulness could relieve craving. Shortly after I quit drinking, I found myself with a sweet tooth for the first time ever. I was having a hard time letting go of my newfound drug of choice: sugar. Out to dinner with friends at a local diner one night, I couldn't stop eyeing the dessert case. I didn't want to order a piece of the berry cream cake, but I felt like I had no choice.

Luckily for me, I had been practicing mindfulness for a few months, and the benefits began to kick in. I tuned in to my thoughts and emotions and started to practice **Focus On Self**. I noticed that the thoughts about wanting the cake just kept looping in on themselves, in an almost comical way. I was able to stop contracting around them and instead just allow them to arise and pass. Then I began to touch into what was happening in my body. There was a strong pressure in my chest. It felt like the physical manifestation of grasping. As I softened around it, the intensity increased for a moment. But as I kept gently bringing mindfulness to the experience, the sensation loosened up, and it actually began to *feel good*. Within a few moments, the craving passed completely, and I skipped the cake.

The experience of being mindful with any craving is no different from the story I just shared. Notice the thoughts and emotions associated with sexual craving. When you feel that urge arise, take a few deep breaths and start to focus on the activity in your mind and the sensations in your body. You'll be amazed at how quickly a craving can pass if you just take those simple steps.

Here is a meditation for working with craving. This is a technique to use when a craving is arising.

the practice

- When you become aware of a craving arising, place your attention on your body.

- Notice and explore the sensations associated with the craving. You may find that they are concentrated in the chest and stomach, but they could be anywhere.

- Begin to pay attention to any expansion or contraction in the sensations.

- When you feel an expansion, label it EXPANSION. When you feel a contraction, label it CONTRACTION. If you are aware of both at the same time you can simply label that BOTH.

- Start to notice how cravings move in waves. They get stronger and then subside.

- Explore the impermanence of craving.

- If you get pulled into thought, just come back to the body.

While you are exploring celibacy this technique will be quite helpful. Take the time to pause with your craving, really exploring the waves of sensation. Learning to pause and hang out with the sensations of craving will not only support your celibacy but also be a great tool for any other cravings you want to get perpective on.

Some say that living a life of celibacy is easier than engaging in romantic relationships and having sex. I have to say I understand this. Being in a relationship is hard. It will bring up the best *and* worst in you, challenging you in ways you might not have imagined beforehand. It is easier, in a sense, to call that part of life off and just focus on your spiritual practice. For many of us, though, that's not an option. I'd rather face the challenge of being a sexual animal head on, ferocious and free. There is a spiritual path that leads to all kinds of awakenings, that traverses right through romantic love, lust, and sex. It's the path of the householder, a path of radical humanity, a path of pleasure and suffering and beauty. I deeply respect the people who choose to dedicate their lives only to waking up and then helping others to do the same. I also respect the people who choose to do the same thing, but down in the village rather than up on the mountain top.

twelve
different strokes

You are a beautiful and remarkably singular creation. There is nothing else quite like you and there never will be. You are one with everything, but you are also unique and rare beyond measure. So it only makes sense that you have your own personal sexual creativity and imagination.

This creative current of sexual desire and fantasy changes and evolves as you do. The more you get conscious, curious, and accepting of your personal sexual twists and kinks, the more fun and depth will be available to you. Making friends with your sexual appetites is the beginning of a spectacular relationship with yourself. Don't wait another day to introduce yourself to your desires and fantasies. You deserve to open up to all of the wonders that your sexual creativity holds for you.

When I began to realize that I didn't have to be ashamed of my sexual fantasies, it felt like being released from a cage. As sex-positive as I've always been, it was hard to fathom that I was the one holding the key to that cage. All those years of hiding aspects of my sexual appetite fell away.

Fantasy Land

I spent a lot of time in fantasy when I was younger. I had a girl-friend who used to shake her head and say to me *you are always off in a fantasy land.* She wasn't talking about a sexy fantasy. She meant that I was always stuck in my thoughts. Obsessing about one thing or another, replaying a fight we had the day before, or just plain not being present. At the time, I had no idea what she meant when she said this. At some point, long after that relationship had ended, my meditation practice showed me exactly what she was referring to. I had been living in a fantasy land in my head.

Before waking up, we are all living in a fantasy. Sometimes we are living in more than one fantasy. There is the fantasy of separation—believing that you are separate from everything else. Once you have had the insight of oneness, you can never fully believe that again. Or there is the fantasy of immortality—that old age, illness, and death will never come for us and those we love. The emphasis on illness and death in certain spiritual traditions is there for a good reason: to wake you up from the fantasy that it's not going to happen to you. Fantasy can be a lifelong companion.

At a smaller level, we are constantly indulging in fantasies, second by second in daily life. Maybe you are telling yourself that you are unlovable because someone you went on a date with hasn't texted you back. Or maybe you are telling yourself that you are a failure after being let go from your job. Those are negative examples; positive fantasies can be just as dangerous. Telling yourself that you are infallible and never make mistakes can lead to an unhealthy cycle of perfectionism. Any story that you tell yourself which assumes a fixed state—where you are either one thing or another—is a fantasy and can lead to suffering.

Until you learn to deconstruct and witness your own thoughts, you won't recognize all of the unhealthy fantasies in your daily life.

Meditation can help facilitate that process. Sexual fantasy, on the other hand, can be healthy and creative. But you won't have the mental energy to spend on sexual fantasy as long as you are continuing to indulge in fantasies in your daily life. So, if you are interested in incorporating fantasy into your sex life, I also recommend taking the time to deconstruct (using your meditation practice) the fantasies that exist in your day-to-day life. That way you'll get the most out of what your imagination cooks up in the bedroom. You can think of this as giving your imagination an oil change. Your meditation practice will remove all the gunk, or really your belief in and attachment to the gunk, leaving the engine of your imagination clean and ready to create some naughty fantasies. What adventures and pleasure are ready to spring from your and your partner's imaginations? As you start to explore, you'll see that the material is endless. This is a place where being able to use your mind, rather than it using you, really comes in handy. The mind is your most important sex organ.

You don't want to get set exclusively on one fantasy or to need fantasy every time to get off. That takes you right back to getting stuck in fantasy and relying on it. Instead, use fantasy as one of the many delicious flavors of good sex. And allow variety into your fantasy life—let it be limitless. Some of the fantasies that surface in your mind might surprise you (and your partners!), and that's great, as long as you both feel comfortable bringing them to life. There may be other fantasies that you are bothered by and judge harshly. You will want to deal with the pesky judgment that arises to try and beat your fantasies down.

Judgment

Judgment and fear make us contract emotionally and mentally, which leads to suffering. What if you were allowed to share all your fantasies with yourself, and maybe with a partner too? What might that open up in you? How might you expand and grow, spiritually and sexually, as a result?

Sharing your fantasies can be uncomfortable. It can be a sensitive thing to talk about your desire for more domination or submission. You may be worried about how your partner will take your fantasy about a threesome. It might feel embarrassing to tell your partner that you want to dress up in a white coat and play doctor. Maybe it feels too uncomfortably intimate to share your wish to explore Tantric sex, or orgasmic meditation. Your mind can convince you that it's too scary to speak your fantasies out loud to your partner.

But you don't have to listen to your mind when it tells you to hide your sexual fantasy land away. You are a creative being, and shutting any aspect of self down is a recipe for suffering. We owe ourselves and our partners the gift of our unique sexual imagination. Allowing for free expression leads us into the mystery that good sex really is. Good sex is not some planned out, sterile activity. It's a flowing, ever-changing activity that can only fully blossom when we open the gates and let it out to play.

Each time you shine the light of awareness on your sexual fantasies, you are knowing yourself more deeply. Don't be surprised if honoring your fantasies in your sex life allows you to honor your healthy fantasies in all regions of your life. You may find that simply being willing to share your fantasy to drink a root beer float while you get head gives a voice to your fantasy of learning to play the piano. When you expand your sexual horizons you expand your life. You may not be ready to share all your fantasies with someone else, and that's okay. Baby steps are still steps in the right direction.

Keep in mind that some fantasies are just that. Fantasies. Just because you have a rape fantasy, as a large number of women do, doesn't in any way mean that you actually want to be raped. It's okay to have violent or taboo fantasies. It's okay to act them out in a safe and consensual way. Your sexuality is yours and there is nothing to judge or be ashamed of.

Here is a writing exercise to help you get started down the path to freeing your fantasies.

—

the practice

- Start with some stream of consciousness writing. Write at least a page of whatever wants to come up. It doesn't have to be related to sex or fantasy.

- Now, write down your self-judgments about your sexuality or sexual fantasies. Keep writing until it's all on the page.

- Write down any time you have felt judged for your sexuality or sexual fantasies.

- Close your eyes, relax from your head to your toes, and say these phrases:

  > I let go of any judgment toward myself about my sexuality or sexual fantasies.

  > I let go of any ways others have judged my sexuality or sexual fantasies.

  > I let go of any resentment toward myself or anyone else for judging me.

  > I deserve to be seen and appreciated for my sexuality and sexual creativity.

- When you have completed the phrases, write down one of your sexual fantasies. Include lots of specific details. Take the time to really flesh out the fantasy.

- If at any time you notice judgment arising, pause and go back to relaxing and saying the previous phrases.

- You can continue with your next fantasy after you have completed the first, or save it for another session.

Once you've had the chance to work with this exercise a few times, try talking to a partner (or friend, therapist, or teacher) about one of your fantasies. You don't have to rush in to anything or pressure yourself. Just take it easy and allow your fantasies to come out of hiding. As you learn to nurture and share your sexual creativity and imagination, your life will take on a special glow. This is the glow of dancing with the beautiful creative mystery of life. It's a dance that will keep changing and delighting you for all of your days.

The Threesome

Having a threesome is a fantasy that a lot of folks have. But a threesome isn't just something to drunkenly stumble into (as many people do). A threesome asks you to be even more present, because there are even more people involved. Being mindful with one person is important, and you have to double that level of mindfulness when you add another person into the mix.

My first threesome involved a lot of Captain Morgan's Spiced Rum and a mattress on the floor. It was fun, sloppy, and we all had a good time. After that, my triad sexual experiences were all heavily supported by the use of alcohol. Sometimes the threesomes were the result of wanting to be physical with someone other than my partner, but not wanting to cheat. I always woke up the next morning feeling a little confused, a little guilty, and a lot hungover. I never really had to deal with the politics of a threesome, and certainly not the complex feelings that can arise, because I was not actually present. Another side effect of being checked out was that I missed out on how fun and sexy it can be to have an extra set of hands in the mix, or to watch your partner exploring another body. Today, I like to show up for everything, including my sex life.

And let me tell you: Fully experiencing a threesome is way better than drunkenly fumbling though one. Bringing mindfulness

good sex tip

I have a lot of people ask me about anal sex. It's an area with a lack of information that some people are curious about. There are two questions that I always get, so I'm going to cover them here:

1 *Isn't it going to be messy?* If you have healthy bowel movements, and clear your bowels before having anal sex, there should be no big mess. There may be a little mess, but it can be easily cleaned up. One thing to never do is put a penis, finger, or toy into a vagina after it's been in an anus. It seems like common sense, but many people end up with UTIs or kidney infections from that mistake.

2 *How do I do it without pain?* One word: lubrication. Lots and lots of lubrication. You also want to "warm up" the anal sphincter—it's a muscle. You can do this with a finger or a toy that's designed for anal play. Always use toys with a flared base. You don't want to get anything stuck up there! Make sure to breathe and relax.

As always, practice safe sex. The tissue of the anus can tear easily, making it easier to contract STIs. Anal play and sex can feel amazing if you are relaxed, warmed up, and lubed up. For my "No butt stuff," straight cis-gender men: having a prostate makes anal play incredibly pleasurable. Don't knock it until you've tried it.

into your new sexual adventures magnifies them. The more you bring your practice into every aspect of your day, the more you have the potential to lead an awakened life. If you get mindful about it, a threesome can be a spiritual path of its own.

There are, however, unique challenges and negotiations involved with bringing a third person into the bedroom. If you are considering inviting someone to join you and your partner, a mindful approach will make all the difference in navigating those challenges. Here are a few tips for making your threesome fantasy a reality that doesn't require a bottle of rum.

Don't "Buy a Puppy"

- Wanting to spice things up is one thing, but trying to fix your relationship by throwing another body at it is another. Whatever needs to be addressed between the two of you will not magically disappear when you see your girlfriend going down on another woman. It might be momentarily forgotten, but it's not a cure.

- Just like buying a puppy isn't a good idea when a relationship is going through a rocky period, neither is group sex. Talk about what you hope to get out of including someone else in your sex life. Notice and discuss if either of you has hopes of it fixing the problems you are experiencing. Most importantly, be honest with yourself. The best way I know to be totally honest with myself is to sit down and get still. Meditation has a way of pushing what is true to the top of your consciousness.

Talk Dirty (and Clearly)

- Before you embark on a threesome, sit down with your partner and talk about what your expectations are. Decide what is off-limits and what is fair play. Come up with a plan of action if one of you starts to get uncomfortable. Moushumi Ghose, MFT, a sex-positive therapist and cohost of the web series *The Sex Talk*, says that when exploring an alternative lifestyle in your relationship, "setting ground rules is key. Things will come up while you are out there 'mixing it up,' so having key words, and advance communication to help ease the situation will make it all the better."

- Power dynamics can be especially important to discuss. While being dominant with your partner might be the norm, it may not be appropriate when someone else is there. Getting spanked in front of someone else could be incredibly hot, but it could also be really embarrassing. If you are inclined to be kinky, decide what stays in the chest under the bed and what comes out before your friend arrives. If having this kind of discussion scares you, you may not be ready to take this step. Practice just talking about it, while mindfully noticing what emotions and thoughts arise, before taking the plunge. It may be that just talking about a threesome is enough for you for now. Just sharing the fantasy of opening your relationship in that way can be really hot. Experiment and greet your experiences with mindful awareness.

Tame the Green-Eyed Monster

- Jealousy has been one of my greatest teachers. That said, if I could never experience it again I would be happy to skip that class. Jealousy can be painful and all-consuming. A meditation practice can help us realize how pointless it is to spend time tangled up in jealous thoughts, but it can be hard to get rid of them completely.

- Jealousy can come up in a threesome, and that's okay. There is nothing wrong with being turned on and jealous at the same time. For some people, jealousy can actually morph into a turn-on. If you notice that feelings of jealousy are arising, don't try to ignore or suppress them. What you resist persists. Instead, allow yourself to have the feelings in your body and notice the thoughts in your head without getting eaten up by them. Focus on your partners, feel your breath, and relax.

- If the feelings don't pass, take a time out and talk about what's going on for you. Don't use this as an opportunity to shut down. Having checked-out sex with one person is bad, and it's even worse with two!

- It's okay to stop or pause while you are having a threesome (or any kind of sex). Remember that consent, including consent with yourself, is a requirement for sex. Don't try to power through jealousy, or any other challenging emotion. Talk to your partners about what is going on, and pull the emergency brake if you need to. When unsure, just go with the slogan *yes means yes* and only move forward if you get a clear yes from yourself and your partners.

Safety First

- Discuss sexual history and practice safe sex with anyone you invite to join you. Period.

Take It All In

- You are having sex with three people! Be there for it. Open your eyes and take it in. Stay with the sensations, tastes, smells, and sounds. Treat this as a meditation. Use **BASIC BODY AWARENESS** if you need some help getting focused. The more open, free, and present you are, the more you will inspire your partners to be the same. Let the experience unfold in its natural way and, as always, don't worry about "getting it right." Take your time to get to know this new body that is mingling with you and your partner.

- If the excitement and newness of the situation speeds you up too much, pause. Settle into your body and breathe. As you breathe, feel how the pleasure moves through your body.

Connect with the other people with you. Use your meditation practice to keep you present and focused on the experience. You may discover new things about yourself and your partner when you expand your sex life in this way. Stay open to all the gifts that your sexuality has to offer. Be brave and gentle, and have fun.

The Mindful Third

- If you are the third in a threesome with a couple, the best-case scenario is that you are in for quite a treat. Worst case? A big drama fest. This is why I always say: communicate, communicate, communicate! It's better to overdo the talking than to wind up in the middle of a naked relationship meltdown. If you have only communicated with one member of the couple, be sure to have a conversation about boundaries and expectations with the other person before meeting up for the grand event. This will save you so much trouble.

- Be honest and clear with yourself about what you are looking for in this sexual interaction. If you are secretly in love with one of the people in the relationship, a threesome is just a plain bad idea. Don't make someone else's relationship a game board for your unrequited love. It won't end well.

- Remember that your feelings and desires matter. Just because you are being invited into a couple's relationship doesn't mean they call all the shots. Ask for what you want and be clear and honest about what you don't.

Quality over Quantity

- There is no rush to live out your threesome fantasy. You don't need to jump at the first opportunity if it's not the right one for you. Just exploring the desire to expand your sex life in this way is a big step. There is a lot to glean emotionally, mentally, and spiritually by simply sitting with what comes up when you consider group sex. What fears arise? What cravings and aversions? Does your body feel relaxed when you think about it, or do you tighten up? Does a specific memory come up, or an insecurity? Give mindful attention to all of that. Get all the psycho-spiritual juice out of just the idea of a threesome before you actually have one. And if you do have one, choose your lovers wisely.

- Don't skimp on the quality of the people you choose to invite into your sexual space. Maybe there is a person who is super cute and would like nothing more than to join you and your partner, but they aren't someone you'd actually want to be friends with. Don't grab the opportunity thinking there won't be another. Wait until someone who is a match becomes available.

The people you interact with, sexually or otherwise, shape your life. That's why I am now very particular about who I love with, work with, and play with. For me it's not enough to trust that a lover will be honest about STIs and aware of the importance of consent. I require mindfulness, kindness, emotional and mental health, light-heartedness, attraction that is not just skin deep, creativity, silliness, and at the very least, a desire to expand spiritually and wake up. And that's the short list. This level of quality isn't just something I want in a lover. I want my friends and colleagues to inspire and elevate those around them. I want the best and I deserve it. And so do you. So whether you are choosing partners for a threesome or choosing your employer, make sure you are reaching for the stars and beyond.

If you want to try a little bondage, invest in actual bondage rope. Don't just make a dash for Home Depot, unless you want rope burn. Bondage rope is strong but soft, making it way more fun to be tied up in knots by your partner. There is also bondage tape, which works great too!

Tie Me Up, Tie Me Down!

Another incredibly common fantasy is to get kinky and explore BDSM (Bondage & Discipline/Domination & Submissions/Sadism & Masochism). The *Fifty Shades of Grey* anthology, while laughably inaccurate when it comes to the kink lifestyle, brought BDSM to the masses. Soccer moms in middle America were introduced to their own secret "naughty girl" fantasies thanks to those books. Kink became something that wasn't just for the leather daddies of San Francisco or the cool tattooed chicks in New York City. People shed the shame they had carried about their fantasy of getting tied up, or being called Sir, and did some online shopping for handcuffs and paddles. Not all of this was due to those silly books, but they certainly didn't hurt Kink from going more mainstream. BDSM done right is all about mindful sex. There is a lot we can all learn (and enjoy) about the kink lifestyle.

In the BDSM community, communication and consent are like the bible in a Christian home. These values can set the stage for some amazing (and quite creative) sex sessions. Negotiating consent and boundaries before entering a BDSM scene is always required. Trust in your partner's capacity to be honest, clear, and mindful make it possible to dive into the wild side with abandon. You don't want to be bound and gagged without some conversation about boundaries first. The crystal-clear communication that is modeled by people well-versed in kink is a skill we should all strive for. The more communication there is, the fewer opportunities there are to cause or experience hurt or harm.

Make It Hurt So Good

Sexual misconduct is taken very seriously with BDSM, and for good reason. This territory can be particularly dangerous if everyone involved isn't operating from a conscious and compassionate place. I love how much the BDSM community honors and respects the philosophy of do no harm (while actually engaging in a lot of consensual harm!). We can all learn from their example.

Because of the intense power play involved in this type of sexual practice, being present and mindful is absolutely necessary. Some of the things you might encounter when exploring bondage, or anything that causes pain, can be triggering. Even if during the sex you are having a ball, sometimes you can feel quite emotionally tender after a session of that kind. This is where the all-important aftercare comes in.

The dominant partner has the pleasure and responsibility of comforting and soothing the submissive after BDSM play. I think that aftercare is a lovely thing to do, even when there are no red, sore bottoms or rope marks on wrists and ankles. Taking care of each other after sex builds a sense of trust, safety, and intimacy. I suggest even creating a post-sex ritual. It can be as simple as cleaning each other up with a soft towel, or always saving time for some cuddling afterward.

The Safe Word

One staple in the world of kink when it comes to communication is a "safe word." If you decide to explore the wild side a bit, make sure to choose one. This is a word you can say if you ever want to quickly put the brakes on a sex act. Sometimes with BDSM, saying things like *No! Please stop! Anything but that!* is part of the fun. So you want to be able to let your partner know if you really want them to stop. Make sure to pick a word that you and your partner will both remember if you need to use it. If you can't come up with anything, just use *Safe Word* as your safe word. It's your responsibility to use your safe word and respect your partner's, without question, should it ever come up.

A question that I get from folks is, *How do I say my safe word if I'm gagged?* First off, I suggest that you only put yourself in that position with someone you know and trust (or a paid professional). Decide beforehand on a signal that can be given as a safe word. It could be that you have access to a strand of small bells, or the ability to move a hand or foot in a distinct way. You could also blink your eyes to communicate that you want to stop. Again, this type of play should only be done when there is a deep trust between partners. Having expert skill in communication and mindfulness will give you the chance to take your fantasy as far as you like.

Even if you aren't planning to get kinky, you may want a safe word anyway. As your sex life expands, some of your boundaries may expand too. Having a quick and effective way to say *I'm feeling uncomfortable and I want to stop* will allow you more freedom and play in your sexual experiences. Of course, just saying *stop* is a perfectly good way to halt the action too. Either way, the clearer you are with your partner moment by moment, the more you can actually let go and surrender to the experience.

Surrendering

Surrendering to your partner and to your sexual fantasies can take you to places you've never even dreamed of. Both creative energy and sexual energy are endless, and where these two meet is a wonderland of intimacy, adventure, and pleasure. The idea of surrendering to someone or something can feel scary—like we are losing our own free will. But in truth, the more we surrender to what is, including our sexuality, the freer we really are. This doesn't mean surrendering to every whim and fancy you have, or surrendering to someone who is not willing to surrender right back.

The spiritual path asks you to surrender again and again to what is. As you awaken, you have no choice but to surrender your personal will each and every time it tries to solidify. There are times you can fight what is for a little while, but not without much suffering. And at the end of the day, you will have to let go of your stubborn preferences, opinions, and desires. You simply must surrender the self in the face of waking up.

Over time you'll get used to this stripping away and you'll even look forward to it. When you feel a great surrender brewing, you'll know that on the other side is another awakening. I believe we are here to wake up. We are here to evolve into nothing and everything. By nothing, I mean the knowing that there is no one self that we get to have or be. By everything, I mean the knowing that you are all and all is you. Awakening to the nondual nature of you and everything else requires a deep, continuing surrender. Some parts of self will struggle against being revealed as fundamentally impermanent and part of the surrounding world. It's quite common for someone to start up a spiritual practice and then run like hell when it starts getting real. I almost cancelled my first meditation retreat because of the resistance that came up in the form of fear and anxiety. Luckily, I had friends who threatened to tie me up, blindfold me, and throw me in the trunk of their car to make sure I got there. Resistance has continued to pop up over the years for me in all kinds of ways (getting lost in a relationship, binging on Netflix, sugar), but these days I usually know it when I see it and I take it as a sign of something good coming soon.

Expect a certain amount of resistance as you traverse this path. Once you start down the path to waking up, awakening will keep coming for you. You have two choices: suffer or surrender.

Safety and trust allow you to surrender to your partner and to your pleasure. Surrendering doesn't necessarily mean submitting. You can be quite dominant sexually and also be fully surrendered to your partner and the creative expression of your sexuality. This sexual surrender is not unlike the spiritual surrender I've been talking about. As you awaken sexually, more will be asked of you and deeper surrenders will be imminent. These surrenders might not be what you think they will be. Your sexuality may surprise you.

thirteen
the deep end

It's time to jump into the deep end of the good sex pool: commitment, open relationships, and jealousy. If you stick it out with a partner for a while, you are likely to come in contact with some version of the above topics. How you choose to handle yourself in these waters will have a lot of influence on how good your sex can be.

There is not a one-size-fits-all when it comes to relationships. We are all incredibly unique creations with the capacity to create incredibly unique relationships. Mindfulness invites you to move toward what is most authentic for you. Your practice can weed out the stale ideas of what a relationship *should* be and bring you into alignment with what it *could* be. Having a radical spiritual practice will make you a delightful and confronting force to be reckoned with for your partners. You will always be moving toward growth, even when it challenges traditional relationship models and roles.

In romantic relationships, partners tend to discuss everything, *up to a point*. Honestly and openly talking to a lover about your commitment desires, your embarrassing jealous feelings, or your interest in exploring non-monogamy can be a daunting task.

Making it even harder, our culture supports sticking your head in the sand when it comes to certain territory.

The topics in this chapter might feel beyond the edge of your comfort level. If that's the case, it's only because we as a culture leave some of these stones unturned. We leave well enough alone and stick to the status quo. But this book isn't for people who aren't at least somewhat willing to peel back the layers and get into the meaty, bloody heart of the matter.

Getting the Commitment You Deserve

I'm at the age where everyone around me is getting married and having kids. Watching this can be very hard for those who want to get married but have not yet met a life-partner, or who are with someone who isn't ready for that kind of commitment. When one partner doesn't want to take the next step (monogamy, moving in, marriage) your sex life can take a major hit. Whoever wants more feels rejected, and whoever doesn't feels pressured. Not a good combo for good sex.

I was recently talking to a friend of mine who wants to marry his girlfriend. He has never had a strong desire to get hitched to anyone before, but he feels like she is the right one and wants to make it official. But much to his disappointment, she doesn't feel the same way just yet. Since that conversation with his girlfriend, their sexual connection has all but vanished. He isn't sure how to move forward. Is this a deal breaker? A reason to leave the relationship immediately? Maybe not. Perhaps wanting more commitment from a significant other (or an employee or an employer, a friend or a family member) is actually an opportunity to make a bigger commitment to ourselves. What if we took that longing for a diamond ring (or a promotion) and turned it in to a longing for a deeper love and understanding of ourselves? Committing to your own life, happiness, and personal growth is a powerful choice.

One way to begin practicing this kind of self-commitment is to be willing to sit with ourselves. Our selves are ever-changing and fluid. Feeling your feelings, instead of resisting them, is saying *Yes* to a proposal from your deepest self. Your deepest self is the part of you that *knows*. The little voice that never leads you astray when you actually listen to it. This part of you is firmly planted in a perspective of love and acceptance. Use **FOCUS ON SELF** to answer this call to self-discovery. You will find that even the sadness and frustration of wanting more commitment from your partner can be a path to awakening.

—

the practice

- Set a timer for five minutes and have a notebook and pen nearby.

- Sit down and relax from your head to your toes.

- Spend the remaining time using **BASIC BREATH AWARENESS** or **REST AND RELAX**.

- After five minutes have passed, write down three activities that you feel passionately about, or even just enjoy.

- For each one, write a few ways you could bring it into your life this week, even in a small way.

- Make sure to do those things this week!

You can also do this with finding a job, completing a project, changing your diet, and so on. Just write down what it is that needs your attention and then a few actions you can take. Keep the actions simple and doable.

A painful situation, such as a case of unrequited commitment, is exactly when your daily meditation practice pays dividends. We practice every day so that when life happens, we are prepared to face it with a present and mindful attitude. Learning to mindfully attend to the feelings of not getting what you want is what allows for self-commitment to occur. This self-commitment can be as scary as committing to a lover or a job. Be gentle and brave as you observe and explore the flow of emotional sensations in your meditation and in action.

Not all of us grew up with adults that could hold space for our fears, sadness, insecurities, or even joys. Some of us were raised by people who couldn't commit to themselves, let alone to us. We now have a chance to create and hold that space for ourselves.

In a sense, committing to yourself is a way to re-parent yourself. As you offer yourself this love and care, life will open up and your inherent joy will expand. Every moment is a new opportunity to commit to knowing ourselves more deeply, and to stay present to our experiences more completely.

Committing to yourself, for better or for worse, for richer or for poorer, in sickness and in health, to love and to cherish from this day forward until death is something you can do every time you stay with an uncomfortable emotion instead of checking Facebook or some other distraction. It's something you can do every time you listen to the small clear voice inside that tells you to take that exciting new job even though you are afraid. It's something you can do every time you sit down on your cushion and do your daily meditation practice. You can practice this commitment every time you have sex and ask for what you want, or choose to open your eyes and see your partner. The commitment you make to yourself every day will create a foundation for a deeper and deeper self-love. You deserve that commitment.

More Than Two

When I was in my early twenties, I lived in a four-story apartment building in Center City, Philadelphia. I lived with my then-boyfriend and our cats in a one bedroom with a loft we built from scratch. Somewhere along the line, I got a friend of mine an apartment in the same building. But this wasn't just any friend. I had been in love with her since I was fifteen when we sat next to each other in English class. I was only at the school for about three months, but she took residence in my heart and we stayed in touch. While there was a mutual attraction, the timing never worked out, and my love remained unrequited. Soon after she moved in to the apartment above ours, the flirtation began. Eventually, we couldn't keep our hands off each other and something had to be done. So we went out one night and drank enough until a threesome with my boyfriend sounded like the best solution for our budding romance. That began my first "open" relationship.

I was with both of them for almost a year. I would stay some nights upstairs with my girlfriend and some nights downstairs with my boyfriend. If this is starting to sound like some kind of free love fantasy, let me dissuade you from that assumption. It was pure hell. She and I were both very young, in our early twenties. My boyfriend was a lot older and probably the sanest out of the three of us, but he was dragged into the muck with us. There were constant fights and tears, terrible boundaries, and a total lack of mindfulness (on my part, anyway). I had no spiritual practice at that time, and I behaved badly. They both wanted more time from me, and I wanted them both to be faithful to me. I threw massive fits if I felt they weren't. Neither of them felt that this was really fair, but my jealousy was so strong that for the most part they figured it wasn't worth stepping outside of our dysfunctional three-way romance.

Eventually, the relationship with the man ended, and the one with the woman followed not long after. The latter was messy. Blood, jail, and restraining-order messy. I once chased her around with a tape recorder while she was drunk. I planned to play it for her the next day. I was just a little off my rocker. We both had a lot of unconscious material that made us both act out in unhealthy ways. I look back on that time and it's hard to believe I was in a situation like that at all.

But, at the same time, I learned a ton, and that experience is part of what makes me who I am today. One thing I learned was that I'm not strictly monogamous. Up until then I just figured I had to be and often ended up cheating. Part of my cheating came from too much drinking and not enough self-love, but some of it came from my genuine desire to connect with more than one partner sexually, romantically, and emotionally. After that first experience with an open relationship it took me a while to try it again. My extreme jealousy, which stemmed from fears of abandonment, prevented me from giving it another shot. Being okay with my partner having sex with someone else, let alone falling in love with someone else, seemed totally impossible. Then meditation came in and made the impossible possible.

The Numbers

I am not promoting open relationships or polyamory, and I understand that it isn't for everyone. Even if you have no interest in exploring polyamory, however, there is still a lot you can learn from those who do.

Out of the roughly five thousand species of mammals (including humans) only three percent are known to have monogamous life partners. Along with us, there are beavers, wolves, and some types of bats. So we *can* be faithful to our partners, but how many of us actually are? Here are some recent stats for you.

Percent of marriages where one or both spouses admit to infidelity, either physical or emotional: 41 percent

Percent of men who admit to committing infidelity in any relationship they've had: 57 percent

Percentage of women who admit to committing infidelity in any relationship they've had: 54 percent[1]

Taking a look at these numbers could lead one to believe that while we are capable of monogamy, it's not always our "natural" proclivity. This doesn't mean that we should all go out and get seven partners tomorrow, but we should be able to talk about options other than monogamy. Often, when this topic comes up, people clam up and don't want to go there. We have a lot of social programming that says: *Hold on tight to your person, and don't let anyone else touch them.* It's totally normal for couples to stop going out with friends sans each other, or to make rules about whom the other can and can't see socially. It's culturally acceptable to lose your mind if you see a text from another woman on your man's phone. Your pals will tell you to "set him straight" and call the other woman a bitch, a slut, a homewrecker. We need to be able to talk about these issues and decide if polyamory might be right for us.

All Kinds of Open

I once had a student call me in a deep state of self-loathing. She had found herself attracted to a woman other than her girlfriend while out of town on a job. The attraction was mutual, and after a few weeks of intense flirting, the two had ended up nearly kissing outside a bar one evening. When she called me, my student hadn't yet told her partner anything and was terrified about what would happen if she did but also didn't want to lie. She felt that something must be fundamentally wrong with her to be attracted to someone else and to have let the flirtation get so far.

The first thing I told her was that there was absolutely nothing "wrong" with her. It is totally normal to be attracted to people other than just your partner. We are human beings with biological drives, sexual urges, and aesthetic sensibilities. When you make a commitment to someone, should you gouge your eyes out, get rid of your sense of smell, and wear a spiked chastity belt? God no. Making a commitment to be monogamous means that you don't do sex acts with anyone else, not that you never feel attraction again. Based on her reaction, I'd say that my reply was a big surprise to her.

Then there was the question of the flirtation, emotional affair, and almost kiss. I expressed to her that it wasn't the acts themselves that were problematic; it was the dishonesty with her partner. I introduced the idea of open relationships to her, explaining that there are many versions, not just the old 1970s swinger model. Some couples agree to talk openly about attractions, some are okay with flirtations, some with kissing only, some allow sex but not dating, and some embrace polyamory—full-on relationships with other people.

What makes any of these relationship models work is total and rigorous honesty. Back in my early twenties, when I was trying this stuff out, I was not capable of that level of honest communication. I couldn't be honest with myself, let alone my two partners; hence the big sloppy mess. I told my student that thanks to years of meditation and various kinds of healing work, I was much closer to the kind of honesty that is required for an open relationship.

good sex tip

Over the years of doing the work I do, people have begun to place me in the category of "sex-positive." I think it's an appropriate placing, and I don't mind it in the least. I'd like a lot more of us to join the sex-positive movement. You can be a Christian soccer mom and be sex-positive. You can be asexual and sex-positive. But just because someone identifies as sex-positive doesn't mean they want to fuck you. Same thing with someone who is poly-amorous, or an ethical slut, or a swinger, or a sex worker, for that matter. Don't assume that sex-positive equates to DTF ("down to fuck"). Being someone who loves sex, whether they have it or not, doesn't make them fair game for anyone's advances.

When alternatives to the traditional relationship are normalized, the sense of shame and self-hatred can slip away. I suggested that she use her mindfulness tools to get clear on how she felt and what she wanted to say to her partner. **FOCUS ON SELF** gave her clarity into past experiences and how they were affecting her in the current relationship. The practice also helped her feel more love and acceptance for herself so that she wasn't going to her partner defeated and ashamed. Instead, she would be able to make amends and then get into a solution.

This allowed her to have an honest and loving conversation with her partner about what had happened. While it was a challenging talk, my student's partner was kind, graceful, and also transparent about her own experiences. It turned out that she too was having the same sense of shame about attractions and flirtations. They used mindfulness techniques to stay present when either of them got overwhelmed or triggered during the conversation. Having that common knowledge of meditation allowed for the conversations to go way beyond the surface, into some beautiful intimacy. In discussing the options, they agreed that it's okay for them to share with each other about their attractions to other people, and that some light flirting was acceptable too. My student reported back to me that they felt closer than ever, and their sex had been off the hook since that chat. They have since gotten married, and both continue to use their practice to fine tune and strengthen their relationship.

Having discussions like the one my student had with her wife require a strong container of mindfulness. It's so easy to get rubbed the wrong way or triggered when delving into these topics with your partner. Knowing how to deconstruct your experience, find acceptance, and nurture compassion can turn a downright terrible conversation into a magical and intimate adventure.

Any version of an open relationship requires black belt communication skills. Every issue in your relationship will surface with a vengeance, as will all your personal unconscious material in regard to sex, love, abandonment, and self-esteem. An open relationship is fierce grace indeed. I think of non-monogamy as an extraordinary path to awakening for the spiritual daredevil. It's not for everyone. But even if that's not your kind of spiritual program, being able to openly discuss all parts of yourself with your partner is a way to have good sex and a good life.

Anything we are resisting or sweeping under the rug will build up. This includes desire for people other than your partner. Being able to name your desire will shrink it down to a manageable size and will cultivate a radical intimacy with your partner. If your attraction to others, your interest in opening your relationship in some way, or anything else is asking to be discussed, do it. Use what you have learned in this book so far to support that action. Lean into your meditation practice and see what wants to be seen.

The Green-Eyed Monster

When I tell someone that I dabble in non-monogamy from time to time, the most common question I get is: *How the heck do you deal with the jealousy?*

Jealousy is quite the thorny beast. Think how many murder/suicides have been committed based on the emotion of jealousy. Or how many people are miserable throughout all of their relationships because of jealousy. At the very least, leaving jealousy unchecked causes you to suffer. That's why it's so important to good sex for you to address your jealousy. Even if it's just a little bit. Even if you call it by another name.

Most are quite sure that while it might be exciting to step out of their relationship for some fun, they would never be able to withstand the tsunami of jealousy when their partner did the same. Working with jealousy requires a lot of self-soothing, almost unshakable honesty, and the ability to see jealousy for what it is. And what is it? Thoughts and emotions.

But here's the thing: Conscious monogamy requires the same qualities and abilities. Conscious monogamy means choosing one day at a time to be with only your partner. It means being willing to have the hard talks like the one my student had with her wife. It means being mindful of what commitment means in your relationship and consistently honoring that. If you commit to real intimacy and honesty with your partner, you will most likely feel jealous at some point. If you can't work with jealousy in a mindful way, it can become a thorn in the side of your relationship.

Here's what Dedeker Winston, relationship coach and author of *The Smart Girl's Guide to Polyamory,* has to say about jealousy:

> Love is not a limited resource. People can't really be given, taken, stolen like treasure, won like a prize, or shared like a toy. Rather than looking outward at what is causing your jealousy, seeking something or someone to blame, take the opportunity to look inward. Examine your doubts, your insecurities, your inner fears, and open up to your partner about these things with vulnerability, not with accusation. Use your jealousy as a jumping-off point for healing yourself and bringing you and your partner closer together.[2]

As she mentions, that green-eyed monster is actually quite useful. It can facilitate healing and intimacy. All that's needed to get started is the willingness to mindfully attend to the experience of jealousy.

The Demon

I had a jealousy problem. It was definitely one of my demons. I have a philosophy that I borrow from a Tibetan Buddhist story when it comes to demons. The story goes something like this.

One night, a Tibetan Buddhist monk named Milarepa left his cave to get some firewood and food. When he returned to his cave it was filled with demons. They were packed in there like evil sardines, making all kinds of horrifying sounds and faces. Milarepa knew enough to understand that these "demons" were simply his mind's projection of the parts of himself he did not love. But nonetheless, he wanted to clear those suckers out, and illusion or not, they were pretty scary. First, he climbed up on a rock and started teaching them Buddhism. We are all one, compassion this, loving kindness that. He figured they would hear the lessons, chill out, and leave. No dice. This really pissed the monk off. He started yelling, throwing his arms around, and ran straight at them. The demons? They just cracked up. Thought it was totally hilarious.

At this point, the monk settled into an unhappy resignation. He told the demons to do whatever they wanted, but that he wasn't going anywhere. At that moment, all but one of the demons vanished. The last demon was the worst of all. Garbage breath, bloody razor claws, a jaw and teeth like a giant piranha. The monk knew that this demon was the part of himself that he most resisted, most disliked. He knew what must be done. With a gentle gait, he walked over to the demon and put his entire head into its nasty, fatal mouth. "Go ahead and eat me," the monk said. In that instant, the demon disappeared, never to be seen again.

That's the long version of my philosophy on demons. You have to just put your head between their teeth and tell them to bite down. Radical acceptance is the best demon killer. I'd add to that story that the monk told the demon he loved it unconditionally. Love and acceptance is all our demons really want.

I knew that jealousy was one of my most vicious demons, and I had a feeling that sticking my head in that mouth would yield huge psychospiritual growth. I knew that underneath my jealousy there was a deep fear of abandonment, and I was ready to heal that wound. I thought that an open relationship could be my chance to meet jealousy head on, armed with my meditation practice. My partner at the time was open to giving this a try, and we started taking baby steps: a threesome here, an online flirtation there. A few months in, my partner met someone. She was exactly his type. I mean *exactly*. Her beauty was quite literally stunning. In addition to her good looks, she was incredibly kind, generous, and wise. He was deeply smitten, and it seemed that my demon wasn't going to take it easy on me.

good sex tip

Curious about the different versions of an open relation-ship? Here's a break down for you:

MONOGAMISH: Mostly monogamous. Some flirting, kiss-ing, or sex with others may be allowed. Often the sexual experiences are shared with each other.

SWINGERS: A couple that has sex with other couples, or with another partner joining them. Generally, there is no sexual activity outside of the relationship unless it is involved in some kind of joint venture.

OPEN RELATIONSHIP: One or both partners can have sex, and sometimes romantic relationships, with other people outside of the relationship.

TRIAD: Three people who choose to be in a relationship together. A person who is interested in dating a couple is sometimes called a "unicorn." There can also be quads and so on.

POLYAMORY: There are many different definitions of polyamory, depending on who you talk to. The main staple of polyamory is that an individual can have multi-ple relationships that are based on love and commitment. Some have a hierarchy, which includes a primary partner, a secondary partner and so on. Others believe that this type of set up is the opposite of polyamory, and that all partners are equally "important."

Over the days that followed, I proceeded to go a little bit crazy. Jealousy took hold and didn't let go. I experienced racing thoughts, overwhelming emotions, and endless tears. I hadn't expected it to be so intense, or so all-consuming. I have a habit of underestimat-ing things like this. But no matter how bad it got, I kept in touch with my intention of healing and awakening. My partner tried to call it all off and close the relationship a number of times. My close friends told me that I should stop torturing myself (and my poor boyfriend who had to deal with my instability). But I knew that the feelings I was having had very little to do with my partner having a sexual relationship with someone else. The level of emotion and the amount of mental activity were all pointing to one thing. Abandonment.

After some years with a dedicated meditation practice, I was good at seeing beneath the surface issues to what was really going on. This time it was obvious. Grown-up Jessica knew that my partner wasn't going to leave me and furthermore was happy that my partner was exploring his sexuality with this other woman. But the little girl part of me was terrified of being abandoned.

I grew up with parents who had a lot on their plates and not a lot of money to put food on our plates. Poverty, neglect, abuse, and alcoholism were part of the backdrop of my childhood. There were many small but significant abandonments, and others that were quite large. I had a well-founded fear that my dad would just disappear one day. After my parents split up, my dad would often threaten my sisters and me that he might leave and never come back. He would do this when he was mad at us, hungover, or not yet drunk enough to get his happy glow. He was not great at paying child support and was often taken to court for being late on the payments. That was one of the reasons he gave for taking off and never coming back.

One day when I was about eleven or twelve, I was snooping in his room. There was a mattress on the floor and piles of newspapers, books, clothes, records and knickknacks everywhere. I was, funny enough, looking for his copy of *The Joy of Sex*. When he was gone I'd sometimes sneak upstairs to take a peek at the pictures. This time, I came across something else: books with names like, *How to Create a New Identity and Disappear Forever.* Stunned, I covered the books back up with a T-shirt and scrambled downstairs. While he never picked up and moved, I was always afraid he would.

That's one story, and I have dozens. Most of us have at least a few experiences with some kind of abandonment that affects us in our romantic relationships. There are demons of all shapes and sizes. My fear of abandonment was one powerful demon, and it was coming right for me via jealousy. I got a good look at it and deconstructed the thoughts and emotions that began to surface about my childhood and teenage years. I could see what my jealousy really was. It was never about what it seemed, but always a symptom of an unhealed wound inside of me. I was ready to heal. I was ready to offer total acceptance to this heartbreak and grief. So I stuck my head into the mouth of the demon.

There was instant relief when I let go in this way. The suffering ceased. I had an awakening around my identification with these past traumas and disappointments. I no longer felt bound to the fear that I would be left alone. I won't say that the demon vanished immediately, or that it's even entirely gone. It took a few months to fully integrate this insight, and I had little flare-ups of jealousy here and there. Childhood wounds can take a lot of work and time to heal completely.

My ability to emotionally connect with my partners grew leaps and bounds as a result of this work. All that fear I had been carrying around had been an armor, and it had finally fallen to the floor. I could risk loving someone because I knew I was safe. Even if someone broke my heart or disappointed me, it wasn't going to be compounded with all the past wounds. The healing of those wounds gave me a kind of joy and playfulness in my sex and romantic life that had always escaped me before. I was lighter. I was free.

An open relationship may seem like an extreme example to some of you. I share the story because it is a testament to what can happen when you are willing to bring your practice into your life. Most people experience some level of jealousy at some point in a relationship. I suggest that this is a chance to awaken more fully and heal more deeply. You don't have to enjoy your demons, but don't run from them either. They are there to give you a life-changing teaching.

fourteen
the sexual phoenix

Please Note: This chapter explores sexual abuse.

Unresolved trauma stands firmly in the way of good sex. It makes people afraid to be present for intimacy and sexual connection. It can cause low sex drive, or unhealthy behaviors with sex. It keeps people from opening their eyes and waking up to the beautiful adventure that sex can be. It makes people check out.

Unresolved trauma is probably the number one obstacle to good sex (and a good life) that I see with my clients. Until beginning the work to heal trauma, there is only so far one can go in growing sexually and spiritually. Trauma is what keeps you stuck in the neural pathways that lead you to dysfunctional relationships and unhealthy patterns. We all have at least a little trauma, and it's all relative. What rolls off the back of one person might deeply traumatize another. So we must gain the tools and support to become aware of, address, and heal unresolved trauma.

Meditation is what first put me in contact with my unresolved trauma. You can use the practices in this book to address your own trauma, but I also recommend getting other help. When it comes to physical, emotional, verbal, or sexual abuse from a partner or from childhood, you want all the help that you can get. You do not have to do this on your own. You deserve loving, mindful, and expert support as you heal.

In this chapter, I will be discussing sexual trauma. If you think reading this may be triggering to you at this time, skip it and come back to it later. This is an important topic, but being gentle with yourself is the priority. Stay in touch with your body and your mind as you read this section. Use **FOCUS ON SELF** to deconstruct your experience and **POSITIVITY BOOST** or **REST AND RELAX** to ground and care for yourself.

Over-Evolved Fear

Fear is actually a very helpful emotion. Without evolving to fear the right things, we never would have made it out of the caves. We may have never made it into the caves to begin with. Fear signals us that there is a threat of danger, allowing us to act before we become roadkill at the hands of a texting driver. A healthy fear response is powerful and efficient.

When a potential threat is detected, the body reacts quickly, beginning with the sensory organs. Our eyes, ears, tongue, nose, and skin register information from our surroundings and send the messages back to our brain. The amygdala, the part of the brain responsible for memory, decision-making, and emotional reactions, is constantly on the lookout for danger. If the danger alarm goes off, the body is launched into a fight or flight response. The heart starts pounding wildly, and our breath gets shallow and quick while our body prepares to either defend itself or run like hell. This system really comes in handy when there is an actual threat. Unfortunately, this type of healthy fear is not the kind we generally experience.

Instead, our fear alarms often go off when we are not actually in physical danger. Do you ever notice your body snapping into a fight/flight/freeze response when your partner gets angry, frustrated, or critical with you? Maybe you start yelling, or jump in your car and head to a friend's house, or just shut down, foggy brained and unable to communicate. How about when you make a mistake at your job? I remember feeling like my skin was on fire whenever I made even a small mistake at work. Experiences like this are not going to kill us, but if we are operating from a place of unhealthy fear, our bodies react as if they will.

Fear can activate other painful emotions. Anger, for instance, will often pop up to mask fear. Jealousy, anxiety, and guilt can be activated by fear as well. When we have experienced traumas, as most of us have, our fears become even more exaggerated. We live in a constant state of posttraumatic stress, always on high alert for danger. We get stuck in a spiral of fear, unable to find a way out.

The world around us sometimes seems to keep that spiral spinning. Turn on the radio, scroll through Facebook, or, god forbid, actually watch the news, and you will be inundated with scary stories. Those stories encourage your fear-based thoughts, and being afraid becomes a habit. We become trapped in a cycle of fear, and we suffer needlessly. Living a fear-based life is living a life of delusion.

Mindfulness gives us everything we need to begin to examine our relationship with fear. Fear is made up of thought and sensation, just like every other emotion. Mindfulness allows us to observe the symptoms of fear from a broader perspective, gaining insight into which fears are actually signaling danger and which are not. Conflicts no longer require all the trouble of a fear response when we can learn the difference between a real threat and some routine discomfort.

Trauma in Action

When we experience fear without processing it fully, it can become trauma. Trauma gets trapped in our bodies and can cause illness and emotional imbalance. We can begin to see the world and the people in it as out to get us. Everything is a possible catastrophe. The more trauma we have stuck in the body, the more scary and dangerous life can seem. We can become trapped in a constant state of high alert, our system on a hair trigger, always ready to react to a threat. A low-level panic can become the backdrop of everyday life. Living with unresolved trauma means living with posttraumatic stress. The symptoms of PTSD include flashbacks, nightmares, and hallucinations. A person with this condition may avoid people or places that remind them of the trauma, leading to isolation. PTSD can also cause sleep problems, outbursts of anger, and difficulty concentrating. Physically, PTSD can cause increased heartbeat and blood pressure, muscle tension, and diarrhea, as well as anxiety and depression. It was helpful for me to be able to label what was happening for me as PTSD. Before I had that concept, I just felt crazy. When trauma is triggered, the body will react as if death is imminent. The heart will furiously start pumping more blood to the major organs, preparing to preserve them. With less blood available, the arms and legs will become cold and tingly. The digestive system might freak out, causing vomiting or diarrhea. You might feel dizzy and confused. Fight/flight/freeze will kick in, and the ancient parts of the brain will be running the show.

You Are Not Your Trauma

There's a saying I like that goes: *If you want to know how your spiritual practice is going, get into a relationship!* A number of years ago, I was feeling pretty enlightened. I had been spending a lot of time meditating, going on retreats, and teaching meditation. I was blissed out and couldn't get attached to a single "problem." Then I met this tall, handsome, charismatic guy and fell madly in love. We had an incredible sexual connection that delighted and confronted me with its intensity. He wasn't "safe" —he wasn't entirely devoted to me. He was strong, independent, and much sought after by a large group of beautiful women. That was all it took to reveal layers of trauma that had been just below the surface of my spiritual bliss. When I felt jealous or criticized in any way, I would launch into a full PTSD response. I would start to shake and get dizzy. My arms and legs would go cold as all the blood rushed to my major organs. My digestive system would go haywire and I'd have violent diarrhea followed by terrible constipation. My heart would beat so hard and fast that my chest would hurt. I would freeze up, and I wouldn't be able to think, let alone speak.

During that time, I realized how much unresolved trauma I had stored in my body, and how I was replaying this trauma through my behaviors in romantic relationships. It was stunning to behold. I had been living my life with a massive emotional wound and I hadn't even been aware of it. Up until starting that relationship, I had been able to avoid my backlog of trauma. I had used drugs, alcohol, and crazy relationships (causing more trauma) at first, and then later I used my meditation practice to focus on other things. The problem there was that I wasn't actually accepting the trauma. Even though I was meditating, I was ignoring it.

I realized that I had been experiencing this sort of PTSD response on and off for as long as I could remember, especially in romantic relationships. But this time, the symptoms were unrelenting. All the spiritual and emotional work I had done over the previous years had made space for the trauma to release. Now that

I could see it clearly, I decided it was time to heal this trauma once and for all. Thus, I began my year of recovery.

In less than a year of targeted work, the symptoms of PTSD had lessened greatly. I could still get a little shaky and foggy from time to time, but it was much less severe. I gained tools to stabilize myself when I felt a trauma response coming on. Sometimes I needed to end a conversation that was triggering me and take a hot shower. As I became more skilled, I was able to become aware of the trigger before it took hold of my body. This allowed me to stay present in a challenging situation, without getting shaky and needing to run to the bathroom.

My partner supported me by helping me recognize when I was unconsciously in a trauma mode. It wasn't easy, but I'm incredibly grateful that the relationship gave me access to those parts of myself. On the other side of all the challenges, our relationship—and our sex—was even better.

Today, I never experience these symptoms of PTSD—a large percentage of my trauma has been resolved. From time to time I need to address a deeper layer of childhood trauma, but it doesn't come up in such an overwhelming way now. I no longer find myself in a freeze mode and haven't for years. Having many more years of meditation and insight to lean on gives me ease and clarity as I continue to heal.

If I was able to do this, you can do it too. You are not your past. You are not your trauma. You may need to make recovery your full-time job for a while. It takes some serious effort to rewire your brain and rebuild your nervous system. You might have to sacrifice things that you'd rather not in order to heal. I had to and I'd do it again. Recovering from unresolved trauma is one of my biggest accomplishments. I went from a life of surviving to a life of thriving. This is possible for you too.

Sexual Trauma

When we have trauma from physical or sexual abuse, a relationship can be like a minefield. All of our triggers are armed and ready to be pulled. Once you are thrust into a trauma response, it can become impossible to communicate or listen clearly. Sex can be filled with fear and shame when we have a history of sexual abuse. That trauma might keep us from being able to enjoy sex and intimacy at all.

Trauma might also keep us in unhealthy relationship patterns, essentially replaying the past with abusive partners. Trying to have a good sex life and a loving relationship while weighed down with trauma can feel like trying to run through Jell-O.

Recovering from sexual trauma is a brave undertaking, but a necessary one, to have the life you truly deserve. Relationships of all kinds are effected when there is unresolved sexual trauma. It can hurt just to get out of bed in the morning, let alone allow someone in emotionally and sexually. Some people can become very shut down sexually, unable to have sex with their partner. The intimacy becomes too triggering, and sexual anorexia feels like a better option. Others become hypersexual or fall into compulsive behavior.

My reaction to sexual trauma was to become hypersexual. From a young age, I was all about sexual exploration. Some of this came from early sexual trauma, and some came from the emotional incest that was going on in some of my primary relationships. Emotional incest is when a parent or guardian looks to a child for emotional support that should be provided by another adult. It can have the same effect, later in life, of actual physical incest. Emotional, or covert, incest is a tricky beast. It's hard to point and say *There! That's it.* There is usually a process of recognition. If you are a survivor of this type of abuse, you deserve to heal too.

I must also say that some of my sexual focus at an early age was just who I am. Years later, after a lot of healing, I still place a high value on sex. It's one of the areas in life that I love to explore and engage. I find sex to be a source of spiritual and creative inspiration and expansion. Years ago, however, all the checked-out sex I was having was fueled by past trauma. I was greatly limited in my romantic relationships and sex life.

Meditation can help us to gently observe and explore the present-day symptoms as well as the past event. By gaining equanimity with the mental and physical experience of trauma, we can begin to release it. We can get to the bottom of our trauma and have an entirely new experience, free from that weight.

Shortly after I started up a daily meditation practice, I started to understand how much sexual trauma was affecting my life. I shared with a mentor that most of my partners throughout my life had been sexual abuse survivors. They were all of the sexual anorexic variety, a frustrating match to my hypersexuality. A mentor suggested that perhaps I was attracted to these people for a reason. Perhaps it was my own unresolved sexual trauma. I told her that I didn't think that what happened to me was sexual abuse, per se. She told me that it didn't matter and that I should start to work on healing myself as if I had sexual trauma.

That work is what led to me starting the first sexually awakened relationship of my life. That work also exposed my trauma fully, which was necessary to start the healing process.

The Little Girl under the Bed

At the beginning of my yearlong trauma recovery, I attended a ten-day meditation retreat. I had been to quite a few by then, but I was new enough into my recovery process to still be having intense experiences quite regularly.

A few days into the retreat, at night, while preparing for bed, I dropped into a state of "lucid waking." I saw with absolute clarity that life was in fact just a dream. The constructs of the dream were thought and emotion. Just as you can become lucid in a dream during sleep, I became lucid in the dream of waking life. I saw that the mystery of what I really am, apart from attachment to thought and emotion, was much vaster and wilder than I had previously understood. It was a swift and vicious blow to the part of me that still hung on to the idea of being a solid and separate self.

Within a few minutes of this awakening, I was struck with an overwhelming sense of dread and terror. I felt as if I would be killed at any moment. Then I began to see visions of demons and monsters tearing my flesh off the bone. Terrified, I jumped onto my single bed and drew my knees to my chest, curling into a ball. I could sense something evil and deadly under the bed, and also in the closet to my right. Along with that, I felt the very strong presence of *something or someone* just behind me, looking over my shoulder (I later learned that this was actually a type of out-of-body experience). I had never in my memory felt fear like this.

I was way too overwhelmed to even try to meditate. Instead, I turned on my phone (a big no no on retreat) and I texted a good friend in my meditation community. He texted a few loving words back, and while I was still incredibly afraid, his words allowed a crack of light into my waking nightmare. Eventually, I fell asleep, knees to my chest all night long.

The next morning, I was still terrified of whatever was under my bed and possibly in my closet. I got dressed and ran from my room to the meditation hall as quickly as I could. What I couldn't run from was the feeling of someone just behind me. It followed me all day and into my room that evening.

I was not actually going insane, though it did feel that way. There was a small percentage of me that knew I wouldn't be killed by monsters. I had at least a pinky toe still hanging on to sanity. At the time, I was somewhat familiar with these types of "peak" meditation experiences. I'd already had some really terrifying hallucinations, as well as some incredibly pleasurable blissed-out visions. I knew how to work with these because I had trusted teachers. Most people I have come across have not had such extreme experiences with meditation, but it does happen. When you have a history of trauma or psychedelic drug use, it becomes more likely that something like this could occur.

After a full day of meditation, I was ready to use my mindfulness tools to deal with this situation. I walked in to my room, closed the door, and said, *Okay. I'm ready to face you.* I placed a chair facing the bed, with the back to the closet. I sat down with my feet mere inches from the bed. The terror began to rise in my gut. I began to employ **FOCUS ON SELF**, tracking the fear by observing the thoughts and emotions that were arising.

As I sat with the fear, it all became a little less overwhelming. Eventually, I began to see a little girl under the bed. It was me as a three-year-old. It hit me that all of the horrifying images were a form of resistance to what this little girl wanted to tell me. When she realized that she had been seen, she began to turn her face inside out, grow fangs, and growl like a small, dangerous beast. I said to her, *I know who you are. You don't need to be afraid of me.* She slowly crawled from under the bed. She said, *I have something to tell you.* I took her on to my lap and said she could tell me anything.

She began to tell me about something that happened to her, to me, when I was three. It was something I had some memory of but had always brushed off as not that big of a deal. When I was three, I was playing with my friend and some older boys she was related to. I remember I was sitting on top of a big spool, something that would have been used for heavy duty wires. One of the boys asked me if I *dared him to put his penis in my vagina.* I was confused, I didn't know what he meant. I remember looking over to my friend and she seemed afraid and was shaking her head, *no.* I had no memory after that. When I was older, my mom told me that I had told her my vagina hurt from the boys. She questioned me about what I meant, and eventually my father had had a talk with them.

Three-year-old me told me, with many tears, that the boys had hurt her. That she was afraid. That they had taken turns. I was horrified and heartbroken to hear her tell me this story, to see her relive the pain and fear that she had experienced. I held her tight in my arms, cried with her, and told her that I loved her so much. I told her I would protect her and keep her safe always. She smiled and let me comfort her. And then, just as fast as this crazy experience started, it ended. She was gone. It was over and a great healing had taken place.

My ability to use meditation, even in a wild situation like that, allowed me to turn what could have just been an awful experience into a transformative one. The trauma of that sexual abuse had been stored inside of me for so many years, affecting my life in big and small ways. It was no surprise that I had been so checked out with sex. Or that I had a history of dating other people with sexual abuse in their past. I had always thought, *Oh, that was nothing. Some people had REAL sexual abuse.* Each time I downplayed that scary experience to myself, I negated that little three-year-old's fear, shame, and sadness. I am so grateful that my meditation practice allowed me to see, hear, and heal that part of me.

The Road to Recovery

That was the beginning of my total dedication to healing my unresolved trauma. That experience with the older boys was just one of the traumas of my life. I grew up in a family that had a long history of trauma. While my parents did their best to break the cycle, they had limited tools and their own unresolved trauma to contend with. By the time I was fourteen, my mom couldn't deal with me and my dad had become my drinking buddy. I was essentially on my own and ended up in countless unsafe and traumatic situations throughout my teens and twenties. After getting sober and starting up a daily meditation practice, I began to unwind all those years of suffering. Traumas like the one I just described began to surface and ask to be healed. There were many tools I used in addition to my meditation practice. I suggest that anyone working through trauma have tons of support, as well as professional help. Therapists, bodyworkers, meditation coaches, and support groups are all good options. One of the most powerful tools for me was Somatic Experiencing.

As I mentioned in Chapter Three, Somatic Experiencing (SE) is a type of therapy developed by Peter Levine,[1] created especially for recovery from trauma. It is gentle, yet quite effective, and can be combined with other forms of therapy as well. Lee Ann Teany, MA, MFT, has this to add about SE work:

> For someone dealing with trauma of any kind, including sexual trauma, the tools of Somatic Experiencing can offer a gentle yet effective modality for healing. I have seen clients go from a constant state of hypervigilance and fight/flight/freeze to a much calmer and more integrated way of living in a relatively short amount of time. To be able to find safety in a body that was traumatized is an important part of SE work. For something as sensitive as sexual trauma, SE is a noninvasive and organic option for recovery.

My SE therapist was like a midwife for my recovery from past trauma. We slowly worked through the layers using the principles of SE. The most important principles for me were resourcing and titration.

Resourcing is the practice of finding a place in your body that feels good or pleasantly grounded and hanging out there while the activation of trauma works its way through. In this way, you are not ignoring the trauma response, but you are also not being overwhelmed by it. You can do a version of this for yourself by practicing **REST AND RELAX** or **POSITIVITY BOOST** when you are working through challenging thoughts and emotions.

Titration is another strategy for managing trauma work. In titration, the therapist helps you to experience only small amounts of the trauma activation, so as not to trigger your PTSD response. Here is a meditation inspired by resourcing and titration that can be done alone. It is helpful, however, to have a guide and/or support system when approaching trauma.

—

the practice

- Sit comfortably and relax from your head to your toes.

- Locate a place in your body that feels relaxed, good, or pleasantly grounded. Focus on that place for a few minutes, returning to it any time you get pulled into thought or uncomfortable sensation. Get curious about this pleasant sensation. This is your resource. You can always return to this.

- Now, bring your attention to any part of the body that feels tense, uncomfortable, or painful. This may also include uncomfortable emotional sensations. Focus on this sensation for a few minutes. Get curious about it. Separate the sensation from the thoughts about the sensation. Feel it purely as sensation.

- Now, return to a place in the body that feels good. Stay with that for a few minutes. Then return to a place that is uncomfortable. And then back to the pleasant sensation.

- You can move back and forth for your whole meditation, spending a few minutes with what feels good and a few with what doesn't. Always finish your meditation with focusing on a pleasant sensation and a few minutes of REST AND RELAX.

After a number of years with a hardcore meditation practice, the slow and gentle work of SE was like a soothing salve. At first I thought it was too slow, too gentle, but it didn't take long until I recognized it was a much better option than powering through. The gentle pace of SE actually makes it a perfect tool for exploring trauma, sexual or otherwise.

Additionally, I did many sessions with bodyworkers, yoga teachers, various healers, and even acting and voice coaches. All of this work, along with my daily meditation practice, proved to be useful for my recovery from trauma. Eventually, though, I needed to let go of all the outward searching for healing and simply allow the healing to happen. You want to be careful that you are not running from one healing method to another, always expecting *this one* to "fix" you. Use trauma recovery modalities as tools, or stepping stones, not as the be-all and end-all. For some people, medication may be helpful during this time as well. That won't "fix" you either, but medication can be a ladder up from the depression and anxiety that comes from trauma. And yes, you can be spiritual and also be on antianxiety or antidepressant medication.

Getting support is vital, but ultimately you hold the keys to your own recovery. You don't need to be fixed. You are not broken.

You are perfect just as you are in this moment. Let that belief be the foundation of your healing work. Surround yourself with people who see you as a whole person, capable and joyful, ready to learn. Know that you are enough and then get to work. As Zen Master Shunryu Suzuki says, "All of you are perfect just as you are and you could use a little improvement."

Fear of Awakening

I mentioned that right before my experience on the meditation retreat began, I was struck with a deep awakening. I fully recognized the dream-like nature of my waking life. I became lucid, so to speak. Terror and overwhelming fear of death is not uncommon in these types of awakening experiences. This is a fear of "ego death." There are parts of self that *do not* want to wake up, or better put, do not want to die.

Waking up means letting go of the way you have always experienced yourself, others, and the world. The cost of waking up is everything. As much as you may be on a spiritual path seeking "enlightenment," there are deep parts of you that have no interest in paying the price. These aspects of self will do whatever they can to keep you from waking up.

Some of the resistance to waking up can come in the form of intense terror. The ego doesn't die easily. When you are approaching a big shift in your perspective of the self, or shall we say the death of the sense of a separate self, terror can arise. Through meditation, you can begin to see that the self is not a solid thing. You can see it rather as a constantly moving activity of thoughts and emotions, none of which signify a whole. There is not one thing, one entity, to call Me.

When you have spent a lifetime thinking that you are a solid and constant thing, this realization can be terrifying. It can put into question everything you think you know. It's called waking up. The ego (the parts of you attached to the idea of a solid self) doesn't want to jump into uncertainty. It wants to be solid and sure. Terror on the cushion is not always just resistance to waking up, however. For some (including me), it can also be a result of unresolved trauma. The fear of ego death can trigger the trauma, and the two get tangled up to form a massive ball of terror. This makes it nearly impossible to let go into the awakening—it's just too terrifying. In this way, unresolved trauma can stand in the way of awakening.

As a child and teenager I was in many violent and dangerous situations. All of that trauma was stored up inside of me. There were times when I could have actually died. My dad's drunk driving alone could have killed me. That fear, while different from the fear of ego death, feels very similar to the human system. So when faced with a big awakening, like the one that preceded the "little girl under the bed" experience, all that trauma was unearthed. Instead of being able to free fall into the lucid waking I was being introduced to, I had to instead negotiate the trauma.

This was one of the big reasons I dedicated myself to healing my trauma. The next time I was given a portal to a new kind of consciousness, I wanted to be free and clear. I wanted to be ready. This proved to be a fruitful endeavor. My awakening expanded with ease as I healed the wounded parts of me. When my meditation practice invited me deeper into the beautiful mystery of reality, I was able to answer the call.

Healing your trauma doesn't just improve your sex life and relationships. This work on self gives you the keys to the kingdom. As you heal, your capacity to awaken expands exponentially. You are birthed into a new kind of existence.

Out of the Flames

Sex, free from the shackles of unresolved trauma, is an entirely new kind of sex. It's a whole new world. Your sex life will grow in ways you could never have imagined. When I was weighted down with the traumas of my life, it was like being stuck in a room. In that room there was only so much intimacy and connection I could have with my partners. I also couldn't have partners that were truly awake to the outside. We needed to live in the same paradigm, the same room, for it to work. Yes, there was still fun and love to be had, but there was a cap on the fun and on the sexual evolution.

Meditation gave me a glimpse of what was outside my trauma-walled room. My practice opened my eyes. As I began to wake up, that wakefulness spread like ivy over my entire life. Being the sexual gal that I am, my sex life was illuminated as well. It was clear to me that in order to allow the awakening to continue to blossom, I needed to heal the trauma. I needed to step out of that room and into the wild, exquisite world of sex without unresolved trauma. And I did. And it is wonderful out here.

When you are no longer engaging sexually from a place of trauma, the shame, fear, and insecurity fall away. You find that it's easy to let go and enjoy sex. You no longer need a few drinks to take the edge off. Your choice of partners expands to include people who you may have never even noticed before. Your sexuality flows through you into your creative life, and you take on a glow. You start to fall in love with life and all the sensual pleasures that it offers. But you are not attached or addicted. Instead, you are gently moving with the natural flow of your authentic sexuality.

There may still be periods when you don't feel all that sexual. There may also be bursts of time when all you want to do is fuck! Keep your meditation practice close throughout the journey. Every step along the way, there are opportunities for deeper insight and more awakening. Your practice will keep you connected to the present moment, helping you detach from the past with ease and skill. Practice mindful sex and avoid drunken sex or sex with people you don't feel totally safe with. By offering yourself this love and mindfulness, you are showing the wounded parts that it's safe to soften and to heal. Trauma is not a life sentence. Your meditation practice, along with the other support that is right for you, will lead you to a new way of living and loving.

fifteen
swim until you can't see shore

This book is meant to be an invitation to a great adventure. It's an adventure that I'm still on and will be until my last breath. From where I'm standing, I can tell you the road spreads out as far as the eye can see and then keeps going. You don't need anything to start out on this journey except a little willingness.

If you like things to be neat and tidy, you'll need to let go of that. This adventure gets dirty at times. If you don't want to question your own beliefs, you'll need to let go of that too. This adventure will make you question everything you thought you knew. If you want to reach the finish line and win the game, guess what? You have to let go of that. There is no finish line. The adventure continues.

If you are ready to begin, you only need to remember that you have always been on this adventure. There's nowhere else that you could have been.

There are a few last things I'd like to share with you. When you earnestly commit yourself to a spiritual practice, there will be certain traps and challenges along the way. I've had my share of experiences with getting stuck and then unstuck in my development. I've also had the honor of helping my students navigate the waters of awakening. Here are some of the most common icebergs and sandbars.

Strong Medicine

As I've already mentioned, meditation is strong medicine, especially techniques such as **FOCUS ON SELF**. Be prepared for your life to change when you begin to deconstruct yourself. For some people, life can get worse before it gets better when they start meditating. Having a trusted teacher can make the ride to awakening much smoother. If you have a history of mental illness or heavy drug use, I highly recommend working with a meditation teacher in conjunction with a mindfulness-based therapist.

Not everyone is going to have dramatic unwanted side effects from meditation, and it's not necessary for spiritual growth. But some of you will, and there is no reason for you to go at it alone. Get a good teacher and find a meditation group to join. Having the direction of a teacher and the support of a community makes all the difference.

To Engage or Not to Engage

There are times that it can feel easier not to engage in your life or your sexuality. It's too scary, takes too much work, or you think you don't deserve it. The truth is that it's not easier to disengage: It's just a habit that you can change. As you bring mindfulness to your sex life and beyond, you will see that engaging is actually the easier and softer way. It takes so much energy to resist waking up and having the amazing sex you deserve. The world is constantly calling you to open your eyes, open your heart, and dive into the mystery. Why resist? Engage with this glorious thing called life. Feel the heartbreak, mingle with the imperfections, merge with the simple splendor. When you choose to engage and make meaning in your sex life, you are saying *yes* to all of life.

Spiritual practice can lead you to a disillusionment with life. It can start to seem that everything is meaningless, even sex. This is a side effect of deeply encountering thought and emotion for what it is: impermanent and nonpersonal. When you understand that all of your egoic experiences are made of nothing but the fluff of thought and emotion, life can become dull. The "trap of meaning-lessness" is one that many folks, including myself, can get stuck on. I spent a good deal of time there before realizing that my feelings of meaninglessness were but another example of thought and emotion becoming personal. This is kind of hilarious to me. A sense of humor is a good antidote to disillusion.

If you find yourself in a brush with meaninglessness, you have a choice. You can choose to disengage from life, deciding it has no meaning. Or you can choose to engage, and make meaning. It's really as simple as that. I suggest the latter choice. Life is so much more fun that way. Exploring your sexuality is but one way to make meaning—there are countless possibilities if you open your heart and your mind.

The Great Bypass

This may come as a surprise, but your spirituality can be used to attempt to *transcend* your life in unhealthy ways. That's called spiritual bypassing. Perhaps you've realized that suffering is optional, so when you encounter your own suffering, you stuff it down with a *Namaste*. Maybe you have had the insight of no self, and now you think you never have to do any personal growth work again because there's *No one there to work on.*

After years of suffering, the equanimity that meditation brought was like a cool compress on my fevered forehead. I had no interest in going back to suffering, and I wanted to float above anything unpleasant forevermore. I had gotten pretty good at deconstructing any emotional or mental experience that I had. I got so good at it, in fact, that I started to use my spiritual practice to bypass my true feelings and issues.

I had a job that was not right for me. It was holding me back from an expansion in my life that wanted to occur. But I was afraid to jump without a net, and so I kept working that job long past when I should have moved on. This was made possible by my spiritual bypassing. I would go through the motions of accepting the discomfort of working there, when in reality I was repressing my true feelings in order to stay at my job.

This can only go on so long before something has to give. In my case, my health got worse, I was grumpy at home, and I started doing a subpar job at work. Eventually, with the help of my partner, friends, and teachers, I was able to see that it was time to stop bypassing my experience, acknowledge my true feelings, and move on.

Spiritually bypassing has all kinds of nasty side effects on your life. It's a kind of dishonesty that makes you feel separate from your fellows. You can become convinced that you're beyond the human realm and have transcended to a higher echelon. You can of course see how this type of attitude would also wreak havoc on your sex life.

Repression does a number on the body. It gets heavy to hold everything you supposedly have already accepted. Each time you jam an emotion down or pretend your thoughts are only of lotus flowers and unicorns, you are adding more weight to that load. Eventually, you will find yourself with knots in your shoulders and an upset stomach.

Bypassing also takes a toll on your emotional and spiritual growth. You may as well drop an anchor right where you are and build a wall around yourself. If you are using your practice to avoid dealing with your issues, you aren't going to get anywhere.

I'm always keeping an eye out for any spiritual bypassing happening with my students, just as my teachers and peers are doing for me. If you find that you, like me, have the tendency to bypass, you'll want to do a daily check in with yourself. Practice **FOCUS ON SELF** and notice what material you are quick to try to "meditate away." Focus on that, without glossing over it or attempting to transcend it. With practice, you will learn to stop bypassing and start experiencing. Then, and only then, can you truly have equanimity and acceptance. With that shift, you will move into a simpler, more grounded, and human kind of awakening.

The Integrated Life

Perhaps you just picked this book up because you wanted to have better sex, more connected lovemaking. You wanted to get off without checking out. If your sex life improves a bit as a result of reading this, I'm happy and I think I've done my job. I do hope, however, that some of you have taken the invitation to start up a daily meditation practice. This is how the real change happens. A dedicated spiritual practice will produce results like nothing else, giving you a whole new capacity for living and loving. This book isn't just about good sex, it's about waking up and having a full life.

Sex is a spiritual path all on its own, if you are willing to bring mindfulness and wakefulness to it. Sex can also be an easy place to go unconscious and become attached. Part of having mindful sex is actually being mindful about your relationship to sex, pleasure, love, and lust. Being dedicated to having good sex doesn't mean having sex all the time. It doesn't mean that our sex life overshadows everything else. Our entire life deserves our time and mindful attention.

The same way a good sex life needs nurturing, so do our friendships, family relationships, career, exercise, service, and spiritual life. Ideally, we are making deposits into all of these accounts on a regular basis. It's to be expected that sometimes we will be more focused on one area than another. It's just important that you are being honest with yourself about this tendency. Every moment is a possible opportunity to find more balance. Getting ultrafocused on any part of life can have some benefits, but you don't want to get attached in an unconscious way.

We can get attached to anything—even spirituality. When I first began a daily practice and started to wake up a bit, meditation was all I wanted to do. I was making plans to live off the grid at a meditation center, talking about meditation nonstop, and meditating for hours a day. It was a special time, and I don't regret it in the least. However, I was not giving attention to the other parts of my life, or to the people I loved who didn't want to discuss peak states of consciousness all the time. I was also spiritually bypassing many things. I had essentially translated my life into that of a "spiritual person," and I was hooked. What I didn't realize is that what awakening calls us to do, as philosopher Ken Wilber says, is transform, not just translate.[1]

Translation vs. Transformation

Translation is a common pitfall when it comes to personal or spiritual growth. It can happen in twelve-step recovery groups, religious groups, and as part of a spiritual or sexual awakening. When you are translating, you are using a group or a set of teachings as a crutch—as something you are depending upon.

swim until you can't see shore

In contrast, transformation is the process of using a group or a set of teachings as one part of a holistic personal transformation. When you transform, you are not dependent or attached to an outside group or a set of teachings. You are *working with* outside resources to change your life and spur an ongoing personal revolution. You may still want the support of a group, religion, or specific spiritual path, but you are not completely dependent on that support.

After a few years of meditating seriously, I had transformed somewhat, but I was also translating. I had translated my unhealthy perfectionist drive to my meditation practice. I *had* to practice every day for hours, talk about, read about, and think about meditation all the time. While this had some clear benefits for a time, it eventually cut my development off at the knees. My life was rather dull and consumed by my practice—I certainly wasn't having good sex at that time. I needed to have a little more life in my spiritual life.

In this case, the poison was the antidote. Meditation and spiritual inquiry led me through the translating phase and into transformation. Good teachers helped as well. Sometimes a translation has to come first, to pave the way for a transformation. You get to decide what is right for you—that is the vehicle of transformation. I always encourage balance in whatever you choose.

The Superiority Complex

It's not at all uncommon for someone who has just realized the benefits of meditation to want to scream it from the rooftops. People who have gotten a taste of awakening can be a bit like evangelicals. God help the families, partners, and friends of someone who just got bit by the meditation bug. In my case, strangers had to watch out too. I had a habit of offering "spiritual insights" to random strangers who seemed to me in need of help. Now I save my guidance for students who want it. Proselytizing isn't actually the worst thing that can happen, though. The worst thing is the self that forms and tells you that you are better than most other people.

This spiritual arrogance is an incredibly common stop along the path to awakening. I've known people who became polyamorous and then decided that anyone who practiced monogamy was lesser. A full sexual awakening would show that no one is lesser than anyone else, because there is no separation. But beliefs are tricky, especially *enlightened* beliefs.

You may notice that once your friends, family, and lovers say *no thanks* to meditation, you will start to feel a little more evolved than they are. You'll perhaps place yourself in another category. A spiritually awakened category. Maybe you feel depressed that you are all on your own up there, high above the rest. Or maybe you'll get high off the assumed power of being so much further ahead at the game of life. Maybe you'll just isolate yourself and practice tons of meditation, grasping at a bigger awakening, trying to *graduate*.

Some people get stuck at this point for a long time. I've always been taught and shared with my students that you should get through the "I'm better than everyone" stage as quickly as possible. It is a very sticky trap indeed, as that spiritual self is a real know-it-all. If you get too stuck, your teachers may not even be able to unstick you. This pedestal of superiority will stand in your way of continuing to awaken if you let it.

Don't let it! Let life knock you off that place above everyone else, and come back down to earth. When you are no longer comparing and judging others, you will begin to see that there is truly no separation between you and them.

If you are having trouble letting go of your arrogant spiritual self, love it. Deconstruct the strands that make that self using

FOCUS ON SELF, and then love every little bit of it. Over time, that self will join the flow of everything else, no longer needing to stand apart.

Chasing the High

A peak meditation state is one of the most enjoyable things a self can experience. When you find yourself relaxed beyond the effects of any drug, and with a mind as quiet as deep space, you will want to stay that way. It's easy to become attached to something that feels good. I've had students that became addicted to peak states in meditation. They chased after trippy experiences the same way a drug addict chases after the next high. Their need to blow their own minds using meditation overshadowed their practice.

When I come across a student like this, I do the same thing that my teachers did for me. I pop their bubble and try to bring them back to earth. Those who are willing to let go of the attachment to the next meditative high are able to move deeper into the waters of awakening. Those who aren't stay just below the surface, not seeing the ocean for the waves. It's the difference between a vertical journey and a horizontal one.

It's absolutely okay to enjoy the blissful and exciting fruits of your practice. Have a good time. Just be willing to accept that you may never have the same experience again. You must greet each meditation, each moment, each breath, as an entirely new arising. Don't get stuck spiritually masturbating, when there is so much more to learn.

Resistance Is Futile

There's nothing much worse than having one foot in and one foot out when it comes to waking up. I see it all the time. Someone will come to my classes religiously for a few months. They will start to feel better. Get better sleep. Have better sex. Feel less stressed at work. Then something will happen. They will start to see the cracks in their reality. They will begin to wake up. And then they will jet away, as fast and far as they can.

It can be scary to wake up. I know this. When my awakening began, my good friend and first teacher Michael Taft sat me down and said, "This is going to destroy your life." He did mean *in a good way*, but not just a good way. It's painful and destabilizing to have your life destroyed. The key is to stick it out until the reconstruction begins. Many people get a glimpse of what's to come and they hit the brakes and *resist*. Doing this will not enable you to un-see what you saw.

Resistance to waking up can come in many forms. Some of the most common are falling asleep every time you meditate, upping your alcohol intake, getting in a dysfunctional relationship, becoming a workaholic, and cutting out the people in your life who will be honest with you. Of course there are endless ways to resist, but it's futile. You will always know that there is another way to live, no matter how hard you try to forget it. Resisting would be like having the best sex of your life and then trying to forget it and going back to boring, checked-out sex. I suggest that you just give in.

If you don't know where to start, try working with **FOCUS ON MIND** to deconstruct the thoughts associated with resistance. You can also use **REST AND RELAX** to literally relax the resistance away. It will often come in the form of a locked jaw, tight shoulders, and a contracted gut. Be gentle with yourself, with no forcing. You will open up and begin to let go soon enough.

Yes, waking up means losing everything in one sense, and that sucks sometimes, but only while you are losing it. You'll find that once you get over the shock, life (and sex!) is so much richer and more satisfying than before.

Kill the Buddha

There is a Buddhist saying that I like a lot: If you see the Buddha on the street, kill him. What I take this to mean is don't get attached to a certain teacher or technique. Be willing to let that attachment die with all the rest. Ultimately, you are your own best teacher.

Whenever I have a student gush to me about how much I've helped them, I immediately take myself off that pedestal. I tell them that while I may be guiding and supporting them, they are the ones actually doing the work. My job as a spiritual teacher is to show my students that they don't *need* me.

You can wake up with a guru and you can wake up without one. As powerful as guru worship can be—I have a guru myself—you are the one who must do the heavy lifting. A teacher or guru can only take you so far.

The Never-Ending Story

Every once in a while, I lead my students through a meditation that can be a little scary. I ask them to imagine being in the ocean, feet on the sandy floor, with the shore nearby. Then I invite them to begin to let go. I tell them it's safe to leave the shore. Slowly, I guide them to swim far out into the salty sea. I always say the phrase, *Swim until you can't see shore.* I can feel the joy and the fear in the room when I offer this phrase. For some, it's an invitation to let go in a way that feels exhilarating. For others, it feels like I am ripping away any sense of safety and solidity.

I understand that fear. Years ago, I would have had the same reaction to a meditation like that. Holding on was all that I knew. I had been hanging on with my bitten-down fingernails since I was just a small child. Letting go was not safe, and I needed to maintain control to survive. But eventually that tight grip didn't work for me anymore. I needed to learn to release control. Meditation gave me a path to letting go—a path that I'm still on, and will be on for the rest of my life.

Ajahn Chah, the teacher of some of my teachers, said, "If you let go a little you will have a little peace; if you let go a lot you will have a lot of peace; if you let go completely you will have complete peace." The unconditional joy and peace that comes from releasing control and trusting is like nothing else. At first, there can be a lot of thinking about *how* to let go. I remember agonizing over it. I would be sitting in meditation, contracted in thought, thinking, *I'm letting go! I'm really letting go!* Once I got a true taste for letting go, I was a lot less dramatic about the whole thing. Life is always giving you more chances to let go and to wake up. You start to realize that letting go completely is something you get to do every day, every second.

Your sexuality is a unique and beautiful creation. You get to embody that creation and express its deepest truths. What a gift and what a responsibility. This precious and impermanent sexuality is yours to express. There will never be another like it, just as there will never be another you. Accept this gift and this responsibility wholeheartedly and reverently. Let your sexuality be a path of creativity, healing, and awakening.

Imagine you are in the ocean. Your feet are buried in the heavy, wet sand. The water is tickling your ankles and shins as the tide comes in and out. You can smell the salt and feel the ocean air kissing your body. You are just a few feet into the water, close to shore. You can hear the soft roll of the waves on the beach. The sun is out and warm on your skin.

It is safe to leave the shore. Imagine yourself swimming far out into the ocean. Your body is strong and sure as you move through the water. You can still see the shore if you look back, a small patch of sand on the horizon. You can see the vast ocean stretching out in front of you, reaching into the unknown.

I invite you to swim until you can't see shore.

sources

Chödrön, Pema, and Emily Hilburn Sell. *Comfortable with Uncertainty: 108 Teachings on Cultivating Fearlessness and Compassion.* Boston: Shambhala, 2004.

Chung, W. S., S. M. Lim, J. H. Yoo, and H. Yoon. "Gender Difference in Brain Activation to Audio-Visual Sexual Stimulation." *International Journal of Impotence Research* 25, no. 4 (2013): 138–42.

Fisher, Helen. "Lust, Attraction, Attachment: Biology and Evolution of the Three Primary Emotion Systems for Mating, Reproduction, and Parenting." *Journal of Sex Education and Therapy* (25) 96–104. Accessed January 13, 2017. www.tandfonline.com/doi/abs/10.1080/01614576.2000.11074334.

Johnson, Kimberly Ann. *The Fourth Trimester: A Postpartum Guide to Healing Your Body, Balancing Your Emotions and Restoring your Vitality.* Boston, MA: Shambhala Publications, 2017.

Levine, Peter A. *Waking the Tiger: Healing Trauma: The Innate Capacity to Transform Overwhelming Experiences.* Berkeley, CA: North Atlantic Books, 1997.

Schnarch, David Morris. *Passionate Marriage: Love, Sex, and Intimacy in Emotionally Committed Relationships.* New York: W. W. Norton, 1997.

Taormino, Tristan. *Pucker Up.* New York: HarperCollins, 2002.

Wilber, Ken. *One Taste: The Journals of Ken Wilber.* Boston: Shambhala, 1999.

Winston, Dedeker. *Smart Girl's Guide to Polyamory: Everything You Need to Know about Open Relationships, Non-Monogamy, and Alternative Love.* New York: W. W. Norton, 2017.

Young, Shinzen. *The Science of Enlightenment: How Meditation Works.* Boulder, CO: Sounds True, 2016.

notes

one

1   David Morris Schnarch, *Passionate Marriage: Love, Sex, and Intimacy in Emotionally Committed Relationships* (New York: W. W. Norton, 1997).

2   Schnarch, *Passionate Marriage*, 267–268.

3   Shinzen Young, *The Science of Enlightenment: How Meditation Works* (Boulder, CO: Sounds True, 2016).

two

1   Young, *The Science of Enlightenment.*

three

1   Peter A. Levine, *Waking the Tiger: Healing Trauma: The Innate Capacity to Transform Overwhelming Experiences* (Berkeley, CA: North Atlantic Books, 1997).

four

1   W. S. Chung et al., "Gender Difference in Brain Activation to Audio-Visual Sexual Stimulation" *International Journal of Impotence Research* (25), 138–42.

six

1   Schnarch, *Passionate Marriage*, 47.

2   Helen Fisher, "Lust, Attraction, Attachment: Biology and Evolution of the Three Primary Emotion Systems for Mating, Reproduction, and Parenting," *Journal of Sex Education and Therapy* (25) 96–104.

3   John Lennon, "Watching the Wheels" from the album *Double Fantasy* (Geffen Records, 1980).

4   Shinzen Young, "Store—How to Increase Satisfaction." Accessed December 19, 2016. www.shinzen.org/store-category/applying-meditation-to-specific-life-issues/how-to-increase-satisfaction/.

seven

1   Pema Chödrön and Emily Hilburn Sell, *Comfortable with Uncertainty: 108 Teachings on Cultivating Fearlessness and Compassion* (Boston: Shambhala, 2004), 207–208.

eight

1   www.imdb.com/title/tt4382552/

2   www.ted.com/talks/brene_brown_on_vulnerability

nine

1   F*ck Yes, "FCK YES | Facebook." FCK YES | Facebook page, accessed December 22, 2016. www.facebook.com/fckyesseries/.

ten

1   Kimberly Ann Johnson, *The Fourth Trimester: A Postpartum Guide to Healing Your Body, Balancing Your Emotions and Restoring Your Vitality* (Boston, MA: Shambhala Publications, 2017).

thirteen

1   Statisticbrain.com, accessed December 22, 2016, www.statisticbrain.com/infidelity-statistics/.

2   Dedeker Winston, *Smart Girl's Guide to Polyamory: Everything You Need to Know about Open Relationships, Non-Monogamy, and Alternative Love* (New York: W. W. Norton, 2017).

fourteen

1   Levine, *Waking the Tiger*, 1997.

fifteen

1   Ken Wilbur, *One Taste: The Journals of Ken Wilber* (Boston: Shambhala, 1999) 25–32.

resources

Skype sessions with me, for individuals and couples: I coach individuals and couples in sexuality, intimacy, and spiritual awakening.

www.yourwildawakening.com

My Meditation Collective in Los Angeles: We're a collective of like-hearted individuals building a grass-roots, secular, mindfulness-based community in Los Angeles. If you're interested in exploring secular spirituality through mindful living and learning and would like to participate in our collective, we invite you to join us.

www.eastsidemindfulness.com

Great spiritual/meditation teachers I love:

Stella De Mont
www.wholebeingalignment.com

Shinzen Young
www.shinzen.org

Adyashanti
www.adyashanti.org

Michael Taft
www.themindfulgeek.com

Open Relationship and Polyamory Coaching:

Dedeker Winston
www.dedekerwinston.com

Ethical Porn: Remember the only good porn is ethical porn.

www.afourchamberedheart.com
www.makelovenotporn.com
www.brightdesire.com
www.pinkwhite.biz
www.oactually.com
www.kink.com

Buddhist Meditation Retreats: Going on retreat is a way to super charge your meditation practice. Here are two popular centers. But there are many more. Google is your friend.

East Coast:

www.dharma.org

West Coast:

https://spiritrock.org

Passionate Marriage Workshops: At the very least I recommend reading this book.

http://passionatemarriage.com

Somatic Experiencing: Life-changing work for anyone with unresolved trauma.

www.somaticexperiencing.com

Fitzmaurice Voicework with Saul Kotzubei: This work was incredibly helpful for me while I was on the path to heal my trauma and have good sex (and a good life).

https://www.voicecoachla.com

Meditation App: This is my favorite meditation app. It's chock full of tons of guided meditations from "the best meditation teachers in the world" including me! This link will give you 2 weeks free.

www.simplehabit.com/redeem/meditatewithjessica

YOU: You are you own best resource, teacher, healer, and guide. It can be important and helpful to have guidance and support, but the answer will ultimately always be within.

Be a lamp unto yourself.
–The Buddha

about the author

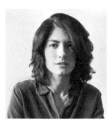

Jessica Graham is a spiritual teacher, actor, sexuality and intimacy coach, and award-winning filmmaker. She has been teaching meditation since 2009. She is a contributing editor of the meditation blog *Deconstructing Yourself,* in which her popular series "Mindful Sex" appears. She cofounded The Eastside Mindfulness Collective, dedicated to exploring secular spirituality through mindful living and learning. Originally from Philadelphia, Graham now lives in Los Angeles with her partner. Visit Graham at yourwildawakening.com.

About North Atlantic Books

North Atlantic Books (NAB) is an independent, nonprofit publisher committed to a bold exploration of the relationships between mind, body, spirit, and nature. Founded in 1974, NAB aims to nurture a holistic view of the arts, sciences, humanities, and healing. To make a donation or to learn more about our books, authors, events, and newsletter, please visit www.northatlanticbooks.com.

North Atlantic Books is the publishing arm of the Society for the Study of Native Arts and Sciences, a 501(c)(3) nonprofit educational organization that promotes cross-cultural perspectives linking scientific, social, and artistic fields. To learn how you can support us, please visit our website.